D0233840

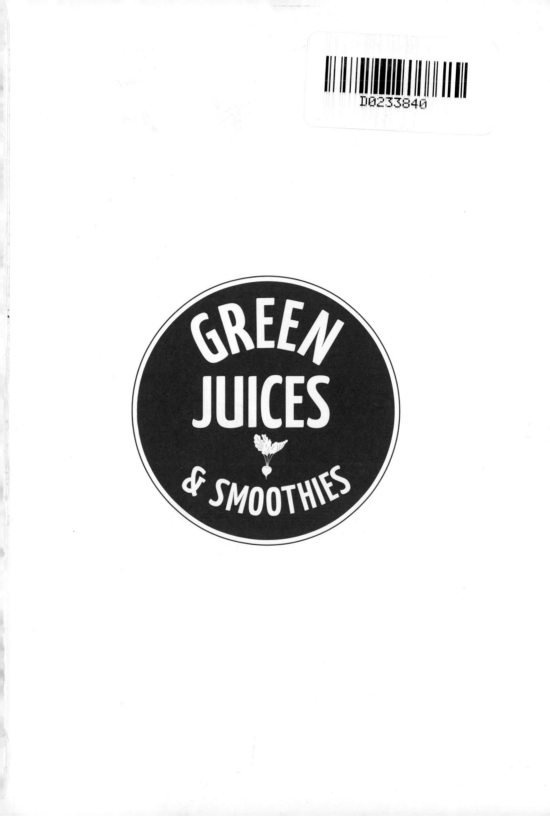

GREEN
JUICES
& SMOOTHIES

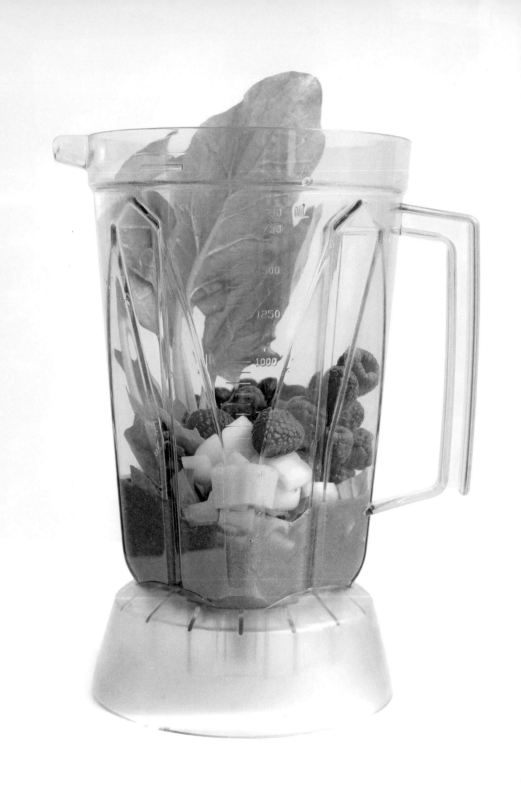

Fern Green

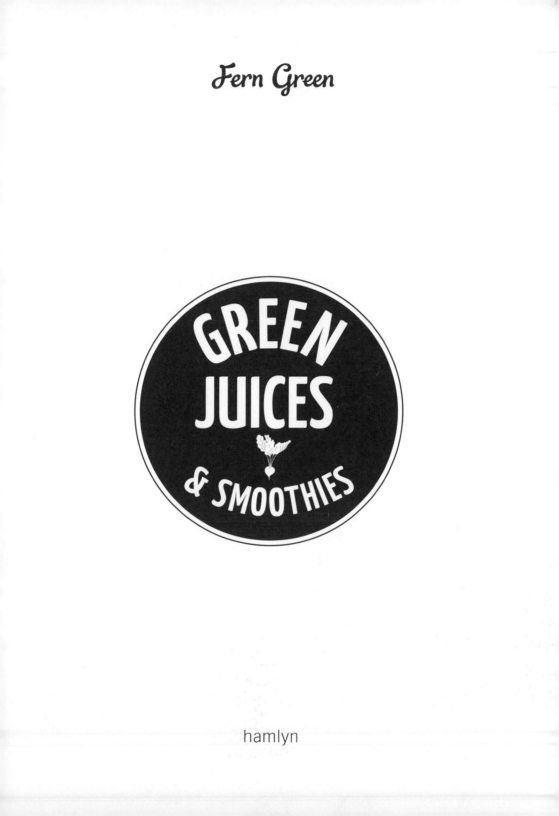

GREEN
JUICES
& SMOOTHIES

hamlyn

CONTENTS

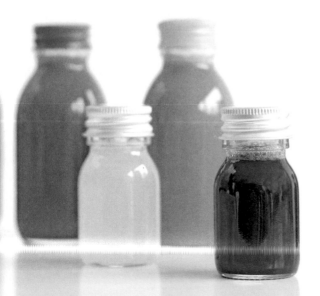
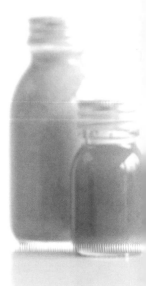

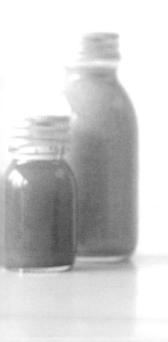
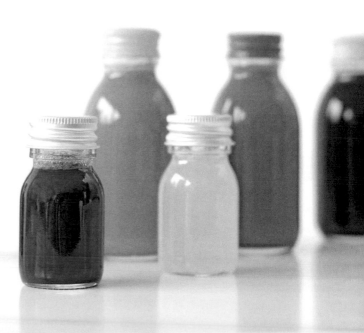

INTRODUCTION

Looking after ourselves

These days, we seem to have a better understanding of how to control disease and the ageing process. We know that it matters what we put into our bodies – we recognise the benefits that can be achieved by eating well and how it affects our energy levels and how we feel about ourselves. Eating healthily gives us a positive outlook on life in general.

We also often hear that cooking can kill healthy enzymes and damages nutrients found in foods, hence the need for quick and easy ways to eat raw food.

Juices and smoothies are a great way to eat all those raw fruits and vegetables in your kitchen. Take a handful of spinach, add an apple or two, throw them into your blender or juicer and away you go – a fun-packed, nutrient-rich green drink! You would have to eat a lot of spinach in a salad to get the same amount of nutrients that you can by juicing.

This book will offer you helpful hints and fantastic recipe ideas to set you up on green drinks for life. Whether you want to lose weight, fight fatigue, combat disease or just be healthier, adding green drinks into your diet will slowly transform your health for the better.

Top 5 green juice benefits

Juices can:

- cleanse and detox your body, as well as balance acid and alkaline levels, helping to prevent disease and heal existing health problems.
- help you to replace your caffeine fix with a natural energy boost.
- benefit kids who perhaps are not that keen on vegetables – you can hide the vegetables in with their favourite fruits.
- help you to diet by giving you energy (from the antioxidants and phytochemicals present) in the form of a healthy snack or a meal replacement.
- help purify your blood because they are packed full of vitamins, enzymes and cholorophyll.

A smoothie or a juice

Smoothies and juices are both very good for you and which you choose to drink is a matter of personal preference. Both are highly nutritious and use raw ingredients, but to make a smoothie, you use a blender, and to make a juice, you use a juicer (see pages 8–9 for advice on equipment).

If you put some fruit and vegetables in your juicer, a great drink full of vitamins and minerals will pour out – one that you can drink in one go and will no doubt give you an energy boost because all the nutrients will enter your bloodstream in a matter of minutes. Juicing is the quickest way of getting healthy greens into your body. The pulp that is left in the juicer (which it's best to empty and clean out straight away) is where the fibre is. Fibre slows down the absorption of nutrients, which would then release slowly into your system.

When making smoothies, this pulp is whizzed up in a blender and broken down into a thick liquid. You can adjust this to your liking by adding water to make it more digestible. Smoothies contain fibre from the fruit and vegetables, which is important to help the body to eliminate waste because it cleans your digestive tract and colon. It's recommended that you sip smoothies because drinking them too fast can cause bloating.

Having just one juice and one smoothie a day can achieve incredible results for your body – just try it.

Green ingredients

When you begin mixing fruit and vegetables, it can be hard to get used to the green taste. There is nothing wrong with this – you will find that you may need to experiment at the beginning as you might crave more

fruit (more sweetness). Add more fruit until you are happy. Most of the recipes in this book are roughly 60:40 vegetable to fruit, and some of them contain less fruit.

Do remember to rotate the greens that you use in your smoothies and juices as variety is key to encouraging all those different nutrients in your body. It also keeps your taste buds interested!

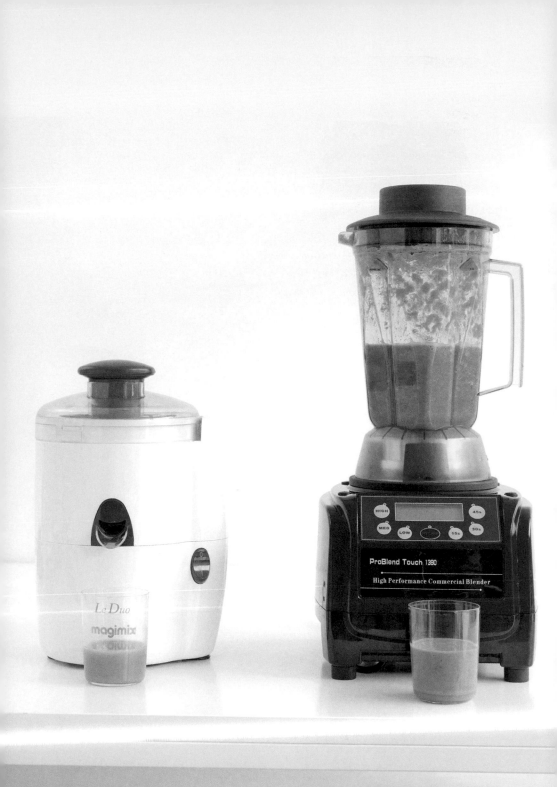

EQUIPMENT

Blenders

Blenders can be a useful tool in the kitchen because not only do they make smoothies, but they can also be used to make other recipes, such as delicious soups and sauces. For these benefits alone, a powerful blender is a very good investment.

You will need to look for one preferably at the 1000W end with high revolutions per minute (RPM) and an advanced cutting action. This will create the smoothest of smoothies, which will ensure easy drinking.

Blenders at the low-price end of the market can tend to burn out quickly, especially if used on a regular basis. You need to set your blender on a low speed to start off with then increase it to blend all the ingredients completely.

The Vitamix or Blendtec blenders are well known and used by many juice and smoothie bars worldwide. Projuice have created a mid-range and a top range blender named The Problender. (The Problender 1390 was used to test the recipes in this book and worked amazingly well.) The most recent blender to come on the market is the Magrini Multi Programme Blender. This is top of the range in terms of price, and is similar to the Vitamix but with more up-to-date controls.

Juicers

There are now many more models of juicers on the market that are easier to clean than earlier models. This seems to be an important point, as cleaning puts some people off juicing. Juicers vary widely in price and come in a variety of styles. The centrifugal juicer, which is relatively cheap, works at a high speed and juices very quickly. Other styles are a masticating juicer or a twin-gear one. These juice a lot more slowly, which reduces the oxidation time of the juice so you can keep it in the refrigerator for longer before it spoils.

A recommended centrifugal juicer is the 'Le Duo' from Magimix. For the best all round juicer, you can try the Omega VRT350s Heavy Duty juicer, which juices at low speed, is really easy to clean and is capable of juicing all sorts of leafy vegetables easily, including wheatgrass.

See page 160 for a list of recommended suppliers.

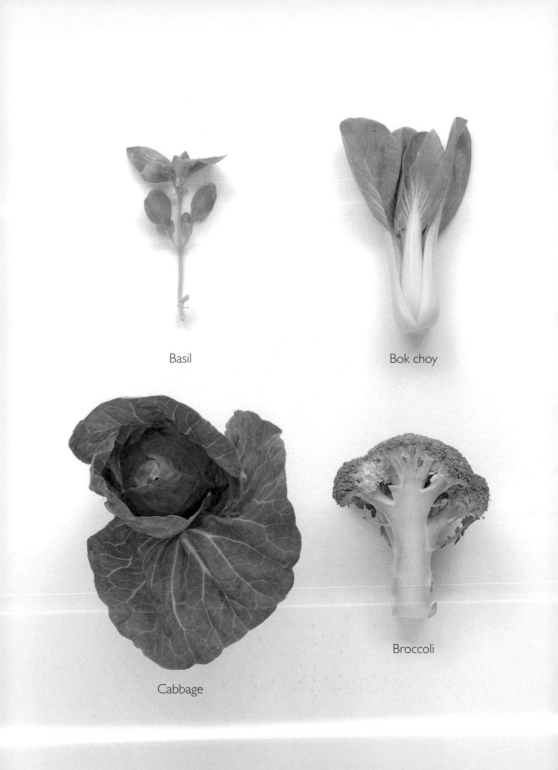

Basil

Bok choy

Cabbage

Broccoli

SUPER GREENS

Greens have many benefits and are full of fantastic nutrients. We all try to include them in our diet, but it can be hard to eat them in large enough quantities for our bodies can make the most of these benefits. Juicing and blending these vegetables means that it is easier to consume much larger quantities than you would if you were eating them.

Also, all these leafy greens have cell walls composed mainly of cellulose, which is very difficult for the body to break down. Juicing and blending leafy greens makes the nutrients easier to absorb, thus increasing the uptake into the body.

Basil

This popular herb is rich in nutrients necessary for cardiovascular health. It is often used as a natural anti-inflammatory and an inhibitor of bacterial growth as it targets the toxins affecting the skin and hair. It can be great for those with inflammatory bowel conditions and arthritis. It's also a good source of vitamin K and contains iron, calcium and vitamin A.

Cabbage

Cruciferous again, as well as a great source of vitamins K and C, cabbages come in all sorts of shapes and sizes, colour and leaf. Don't forget the Brussel sprout comes under this category – it's just a tiny version of a cabbage. Cabbage juice can help prevent or cure stomach ulcers because of its fantastic anti-inflammatory properties.

Bok choy

Bok choy or pak choy, as it is sometimes known, is a leafy Chinese cabbage, which is one of those cancer-fighting cruciferous greens. One head of bok choy contains a very high amount of vitamin K, almost half your recommended daily amount. It is a very light leafy cabbage, easy to pack in your blender. It's also a good source of antioxidants and beta-carotene, which is good for your eyes.

Broccoli

The king vegetable of the cancer-fighting cruciferous family, broccoli also combats diabetes, Alzheimer's, heart disease, arthritis and more. This green floret vegetable can thicken up your smoothies, so you may need to add extra water, but remember you can use the stems too. It also contains vitamins C, K and A as well as folate and fibre.

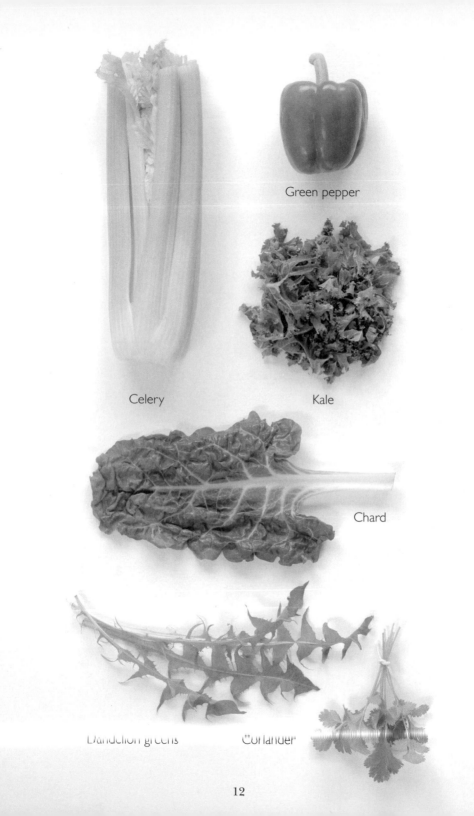

Green pepper

Celery

Kale

Chard

Dandelion greens

Coriander

Celery

Celery has cooling properties that help maintain normal body temperature. It contains minerals that regulate the blood's pH levels and neutralise acidity. Part of the same family as fennel and parsley, it gives drinks a slightly salty taste. It can be hard to break down its stringiness even in a powerful blender but is great for juicing.

Chard

This leafy vegetable is commonly referred to as 'greens'. Coming in an array of different varieties (rainbow, Swiss, red, golden and white) this dense vegetable is great to blend. Full of vitamins A, C and K, it is known to regulate blood sugar levels and provide anti-inflammatory benefits due to its high phytonutrient content.

Dandelion greens

Rich in both vitamins A and K, dandelion greens are known to have a purifying effect on the blood and liver. A rather bitter green, these greens are best combined in juices and smoothies with other green vegetables or sweet fruits.

Green pepper

Juicy, crunchy green peppers are silicone-rich and have been shown to improve skin complexion. This vegetable is also a great source of potassium, which balances the fluids and minerals in your body to regulate blood pressure.

Kale

Another member of the cruciferous family, kale is a powerful weapon against bladder, breast, colon, ovary and prostate cancer. It is rich in omega-3 fatty acids, treating arthritis and calming inflammation. With more calcium per calorie than milk, kale is great for healthy bones. The waxy textured variety can be tough, so keep blending until the chunks go away.

Coriander

This powerful natural cleansing agent has chemical compounds, which bind with toxic metals and loosens them from the tissue. This fragrant herb also contains anti-anxiety properties, relieves intestinal gas, aids digestion, calms inflammation and lowers blood sugar and LDL cholesterol.

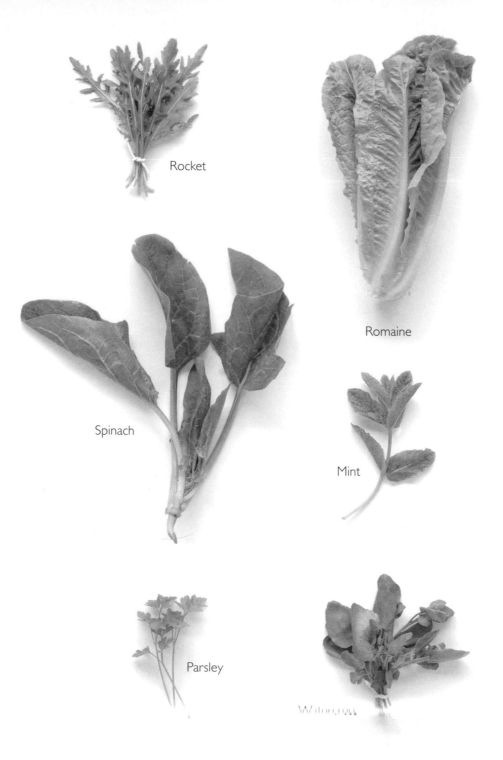

Rocket

Romaine

Spinach

Mint

Parsley

Watercress

Rocket

This peppery, oak-shaped salad leaf, whose flavour is reminiscent of mustard, is part of the cruciferous family of vegetables, making this a potent anti-cancer food. It is also a natural aphrodisiac, aiding digestion and clearing the mind as well as being rich in calcium, vitamins A, C and K and potassium.

Spinach

Spinach is mild in flavour and rich in vitamins and minerals, including A, C, B2, B6, E, manganese, folate, magnesium, iron, calcium and potassium. But it does contain oxalic acid, which can combine with metals in the body and irritate the kidneys, so don't use it in every drink. Spinach helps the digestive system and is also known to promote healthy skin and bones with all the vitamins, and also stave off hunger to aid weight loss.

Parsley

This common herb can neutralise some carcinogens and is a great source of folic acid. It promotes carbohydrate metabolism, aiding weight loss and detoxing the body. It can be stored in your refrigerator for several days after picking and is good at bringing out other flavours in your smoothies, such as tomatoes and celery.

Romaine

Nourish your adrenal cortex with a romaine lettuce or two! This nutritious green leaf lettuce keeps your body in balance and supports your body's natural detoxification process. High in fibre, romaine will clean your digestive tract and strengthen your muscles and heart. A great ingredient to add to any smoothie.

Mint

Giving any drink a burst of refreshment with its flavour, mint helps relax the body and mind. Calming inflammation and aiding digestion, it also has been known to reduce headaches and nausea while alleviating mental stress.

Watercress

Spicy watercress contains vitamins A, C and beta-carotene and has been known to reduce DNA damage in white blood cells. It is also a great green to add to your smoothies to pick things up a bit and to get the blood pumping round your body.

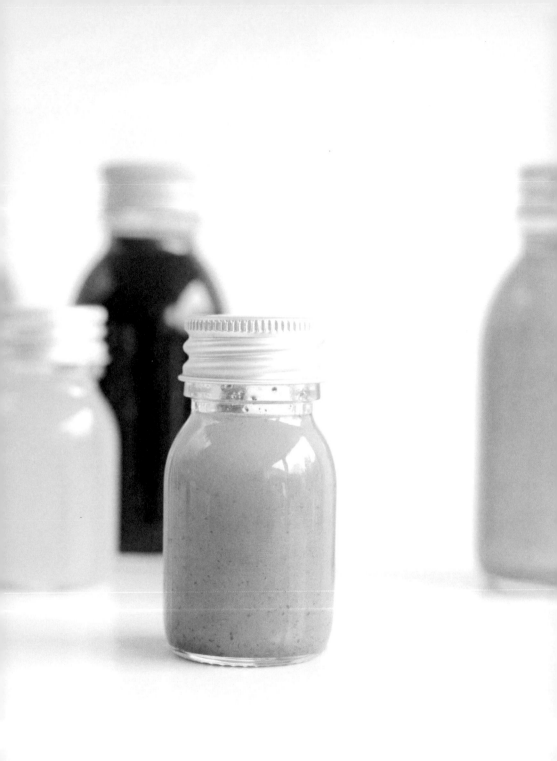

AN EASY DETOX PLAN

We spend an enormous amount of energy on the constant strain of digestion. When we stop eating solid food, our organs are no longer tied up, and all that blood and energy is free to move to the brain, the skin, the liver and so on, giving our body a holiday, if you like. We can now turn to neglected issues in our bodies, remove toxins and ultimately have a rest. All the while, you are flooding yourself with over 5kg of organic raw produce.

BEFORE

When you decide to do a detox plan and give your body that holiday it needs, help yourself by cutting out some things a few days before, notably caffeine, alcohol, nicotine, refined sugar, animal products and wheat. If you spend a few days eating raw foods, broths, juices and smoothies and drinking lots of water, it will lead to a more comfortable cleanse.

DURING

Try drinking the juices at least every one to two hours so your body has a constant drip of nutrients. Continue to drink water or herbal teas. It's also a good idea to keep warm as you may feel a little cooler while detoxing. Give yourself time and space to rest, as your body will need this for all the healing that is going on below the surface. Once you have gone through the first big detox days and are drenched in live nutrients, you will experience a sharp clarity, a grounded calm, a sense of weightlessness and a natural high from within. Sleep will come easily and deep, getting out of bed will feel effortless and the days in between will flow. You will be charged on revived excitement and stamina. Your skin will glow, your eyes will shine, your body's weight will balance and you will be buzzing with health.

AFTER

Coming off the detox plan properly is important. On the first day, it is best to just reintroduce soups and smoothies. In the few days that follow, avoid the same items that you did before the detox and introduce them slowly back into your diet.

Please do not try this detox plan if you are under 16, pregnant or breastfeeding, have any existing health conditions or use prescription drugs. Always consult your doctor first if you're in any doubt.

YOUR SEVEN-DAY GREEN DETOX JUICE PLAN

This plan shows how much juice and smoothie you should consume each day. The juices make up to 300ml and the smoothies make up to 700ml depending on how much water you like to add when blending to your desired consistency. This plan is very easy to use – you drink one recipe quantity of a juice and one recipe quantity of a smoothie each day. You can make each day's drinks in the morning and store them in the refrigerator until you're ready to drink them.

....

1 DAY ONE
    Summer fresh juice (see pages 32–3)
    Strawberry joy smoothie (see pages 72–3)

BREAKFAST	300ml Summer fresh juice
MID-MORNING	150ml Strawberry joy smoothie
LUNCH	200ml Strawberry joy smoothie
MID-AFTERNOON	150ml Strawberry joy smoothie
EVENING MEAL	200ml Strawberry joy smoothie

....

2 DAY TWO
    Green fibre juice (see pages 28–9)
    Alkaliner smoothie (see pages 86–7)
    + Ginger shot (see pages 144–5)

BREAKFAST	300ml Green fibre juice
MID-MORNING	150ml Alkaliner smoothie
LUNCH	200ml Alkaliner smoothie
MID-AFTERNOON	150ml Alkaliner smoothie
EVENING MEAL	200ml Alkaliner smoothie

Extra shot when you feel like it: Ginger

....

3 DAY THREE
    Green rocket tonic juice (see pages 22–3)
    Watermelon smoothie (see pages 114–15)

BREAKFAST	300ml Green rocket tonic juice
MID-MORNING	150ml Watermelon smoothie
LUNCH	200ml Watermelon smoothie
MID-AFTERNOON	150ml Watermelon smoothie
EVENING MEAL	200ml Watermelon smoothie

4 **DAY FOUR**   **Dandelion tonic juice** (see pages 24–5)
                                     Goji tangerine smoothie (see pages 124–5)

BREAKFAST	300ml Dandelion tonic juice
MID-MORNING	150ml Goji tangerine smoothie
LUNCH	200ml Goji tangerine smoothie
MID-AFTERNOON	150ml Goji tangerine smoothie
EVENING MEAL	200ml Goji tangerine smoothie

5 **DAY FIVE**   **Grass energy juice** (see pages 30–1)
                                       Avocado smoothie (see pages 92–3)
                                       + Almond milk (see pages 150–1)

BREAKFAST	300ml Grass energy juice
MID-MORNING	150ml Avocado smoothie
LUNCH	200ml Avocado smoothie
MID-AFTERNOON	150ml Avocado smoothie
EVENING MEAL	200ml Avocado smoothie

Extra milk when you feel like it: Almond milk without the sweetener (agave syrup)

6 **DAY SIX**   **Beetroot beauty juice** (see pages 36–7)
                                     Aloe leaf smoothie (see pages 122–3)

BREAKFAST	300ml Beetroot beauty juice
MID-MORNING	150ml Aloe leaf smoothie
LUNCH	200ml Aloe leaf smoothie
MID-AFTERNOON	150ml Aloe leaf smoothie
EVENING MEAL	200ml Aloe leaf smoothie

7 **DAY SEVEN**   **Cleanser juice** (see pages 64–5)
                                     Blueberry chia smoothie (see pages 134–5)

BREAKFAST	300ml Cleanser juice
MID-MORNING	150ml Blueberry chia smoothie
LUNCH	200ml Blueberry chia smoothie
MID-AFTERNOON	150ml Blueberry chia smoothie
EVENING MEAL	200ml Blueberry chia smoothie

JUICES

Juicing is very quick and easy. All you need are your juicer, a sharp knife and a chopping board. Remember to peel your citrus fruits if your juicer doesn't have a citrus juicing attachment. Also, make sure that the jug that you use is under the right outlet. Most of these recipes produce 200–300ml of liquid.

GREEN ROCKET TONIC
Savoury spice

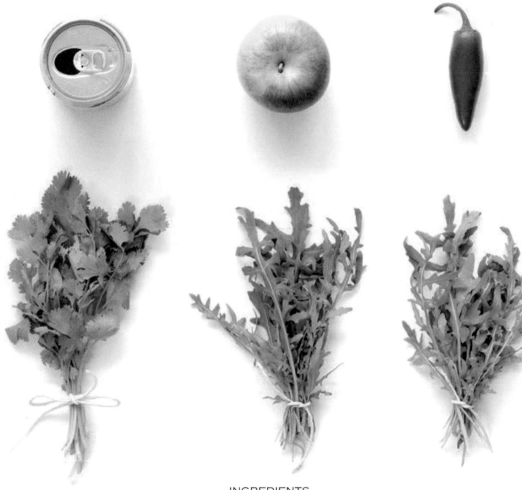

INGREDIENTS

½ can of coconut water • 2 handfuls of rocket

1 apple • A small bunch of coriander

1 jalapeño pepper (or adjust according to taste)

———

Pour the coconut water into a glass. Juice all the other
ingredients and add to the glass. Stir, then drink

This juice is a natural aphrodisiac, aiding digestion
and helping to clear the mind.

(De) *Detoxifying* (I) *Immunising* (BS) *Body stimulating*

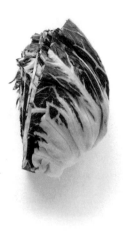

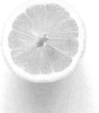

INGREDIENTS

A pinch of cayenne pepper • ¼ radicchio

A handful of dandelion greens

A thumb of ginger • A squeeze of lemon

Add the cayenne pepper to the glass. Juice the radicchio, dandelion
greens and the ginger, and add to the glass. Slice the lemon and
squeeze into the glass. Give the juice a little stir and drink.

This juice is rich in chlorophyll, which helps to clean your vital organs as well as giving your skin a boost.

C Cleansing Di Diuretic MB Metabolism boosting

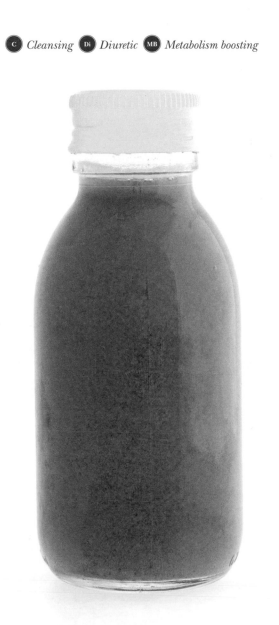

INSALATA
Savoury

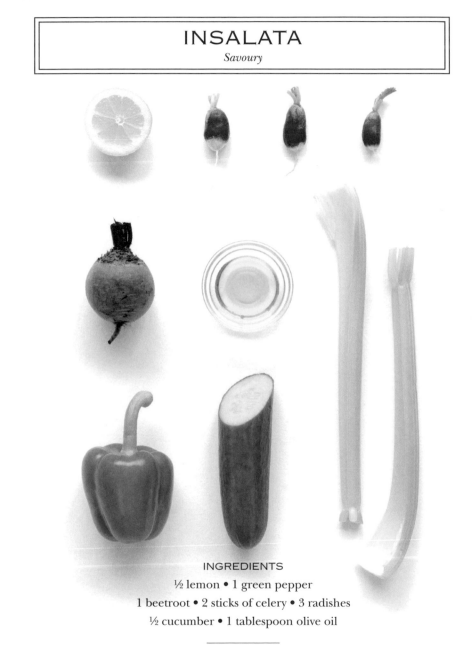

INGREDIENTS
½ lemon • 1 green pepper
1 beetroot • 2 sticks of celery • 3 radishes
½ cucumber • 1 tablespoon olive oil

Juice the lemon first using the citrus attachment if you have one.
Otherwise peel the lemon and juice along with the rest of the
vegetables. Add the olive oil to the glass and stir.

This juice will not only boost your metabolism, but is also high in potassium, which helps lower blood pressure.

I *Immunising* **BS** *Body stimulating* **A** *Alkalising*

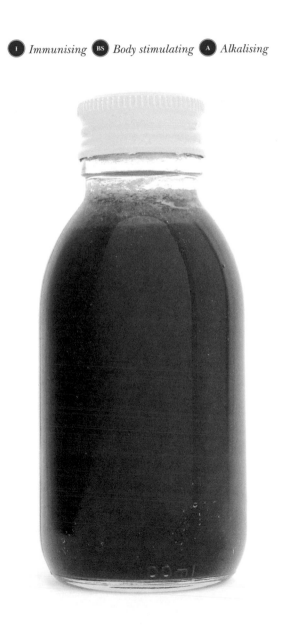

GREEN FIBRE
Savoury

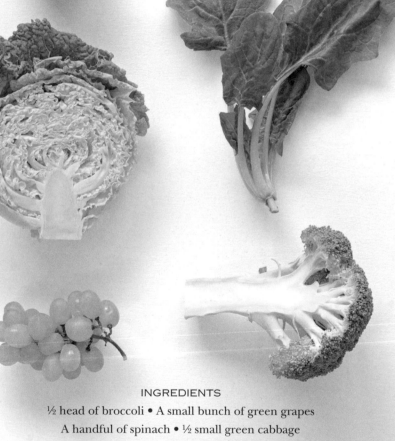

INGREDIENTS
½ head of broccoli • A small bunch of green grapes
A handful of spinach • ½ small green cabbage
1 apple

Juice all the ingredients.

This juice contains a large amount of vitamin C and is loaded with antioxidants to fight off diseases.

DE *Digestion enhancing* **SE** *Skin enhancing* **BN** *Blood nourishing*

GRASS ENERGY

Savoury ... only just!

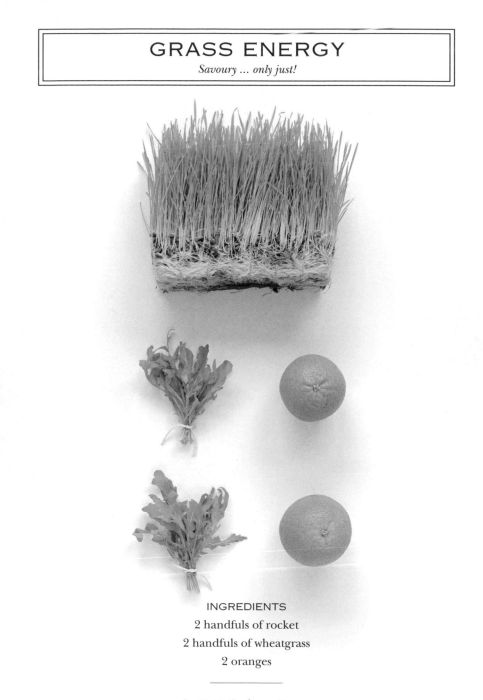

INGREDIENTS

2 handfuls of rocket

2 handfuls of wheatgrass

2 oranges

Juice all the ingredients.

High in vitamins A, C and K, this juice is an effective stimulant, providing amazing energy and power for the whole body.

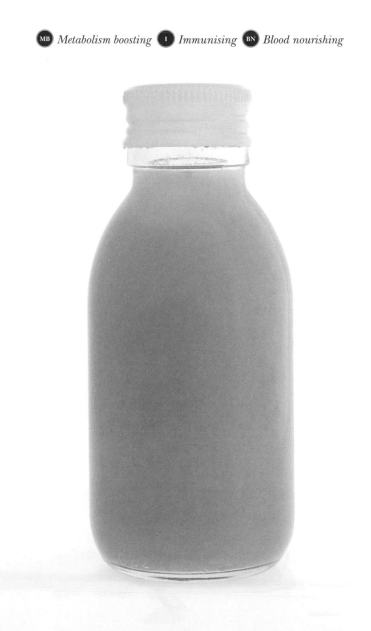 Metabolism boosting ● Immunising ● Blood nourishing

SUMMER FRESH
Savoury & thirst quenching

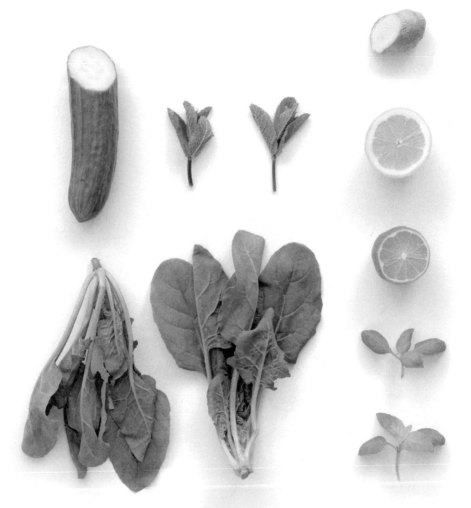

INGREDIENTS
2 sprigs of basil • 2 sprigs of mint • 2 handfuls of spinach
½ cucumber • ½ lemon • ½ lime
A thumb of ginger

Juice all the ingredients. Add a red apple if you find it too sour.

This is a delicious juice, which is rich in vitamins A and K.

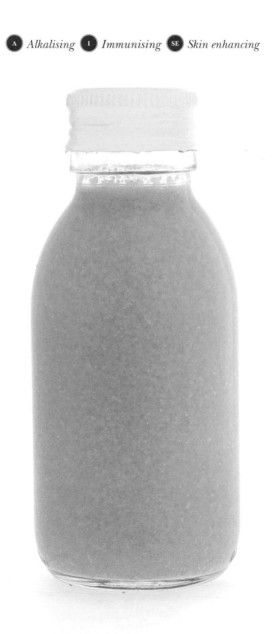

A *Alkalising*　**I** *Immunising*　**SE** *Skin enhancing*

GREEN PEPPER
Savoury spice

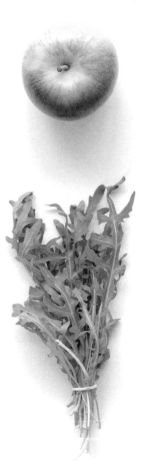

INGREDIENTS
3 jalapeño peppers • 1 green pepper
½ cucumber • 2 handfuls of rocket
1 apple

Juice all the ingredients.

This juice is full of immune-boosting nutrients and is rich in calcium, vitamin C and iron.

MB *Metabolism booster* **AI** *Anti-inflammatory* **BN** *Blood nourishing*

BEETROOT BEAUTY

Slightly sweet

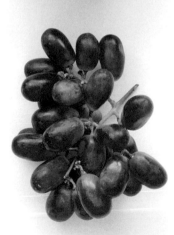

INGREDIENTS

2 beetroots • 1 pomegranate

A bunch of red grapes

A squeeze of lemon

Extract the seeds from your pomegranate and juice. Juice the
rest of the ingredients. Stir together, then drink.

Half of your recommended daily intake of vitamin C
is packed into this juice.

FF *Fat flushing* **De** *Detoxifying* **SC** *Skin cleansing*

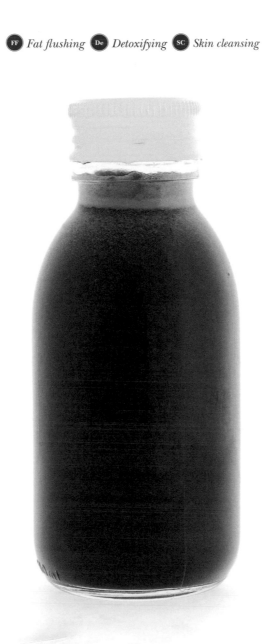

HEALER
Savoury

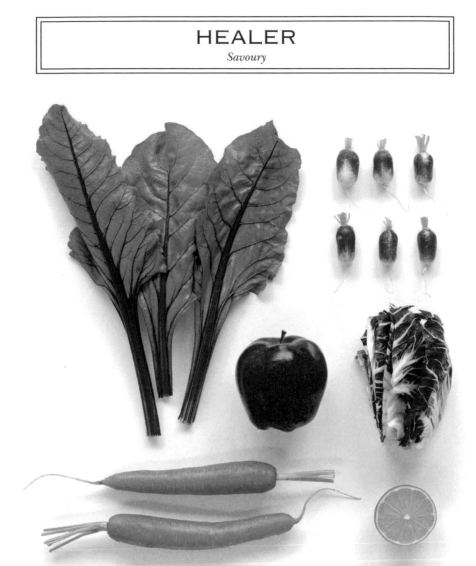

INGREDIENTS
¼ radicchio • 6 radishes

1 red apple • A small bunch of chard

½ lime • 2 carrots

Juice all the ingredients.

This invigorating juice is great for the skin and the brain, and is rich in riboflavin and vitamin B-6.

I Immunising *AO* Anti-oxidising *A* Alkalising

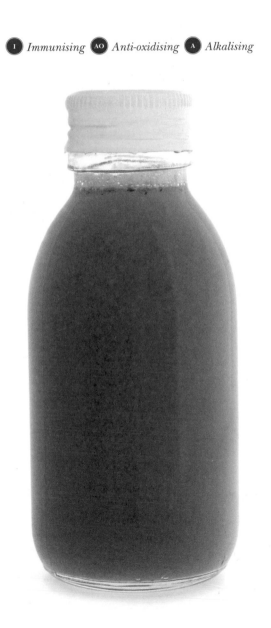

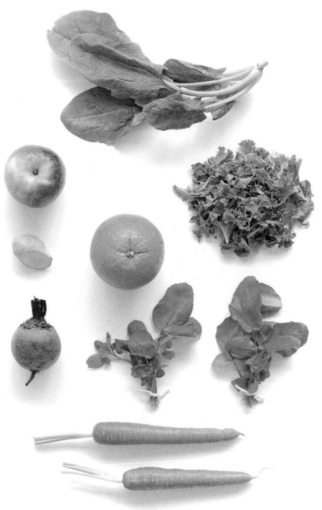

INGREDIENTS

A handful of kale • 2 handfuls of watercress
1 beetroot • A thumb of ginger • 2 small carrots
A handful of spinach • 1 apple • 1 orange

Juice all the ingredients.

This juice is full of vitamins and minerals, including high quantities of folic acid.

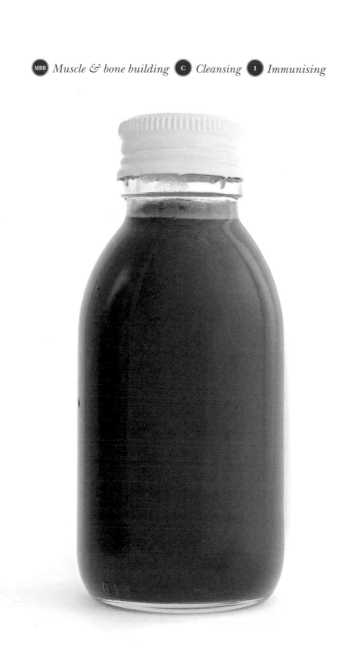 Muscle & bone building Cleansing Immunising

BRUSSELS
Slightly sweet

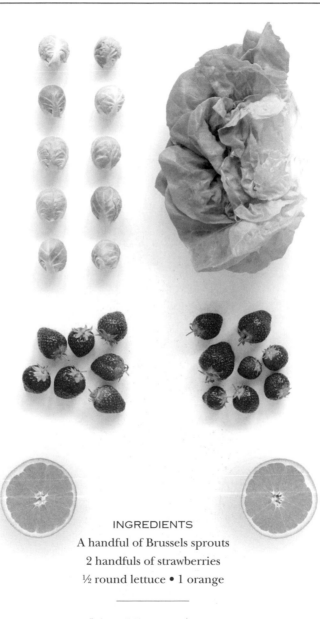

INGREDIENTS
A handful of Brussels sprouts
2 handfuls of strawberries
½ round lettuce • 1 orange

Juice all the ingredients

High in vitamin C, this juice helps you stave off hunger.

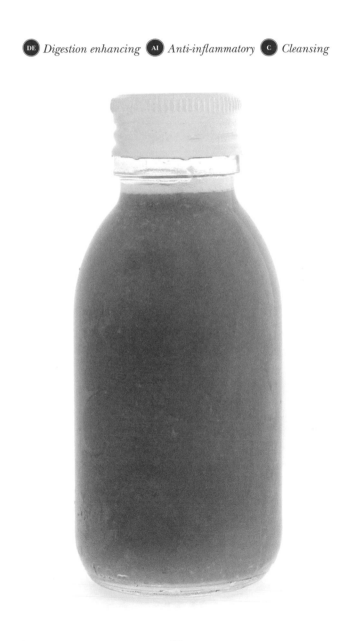

DE *Digestion enhancing* **AI** *Anti-inflammatory* **C** *Cleansing*

BRAIN JUICE
Slightly sweet

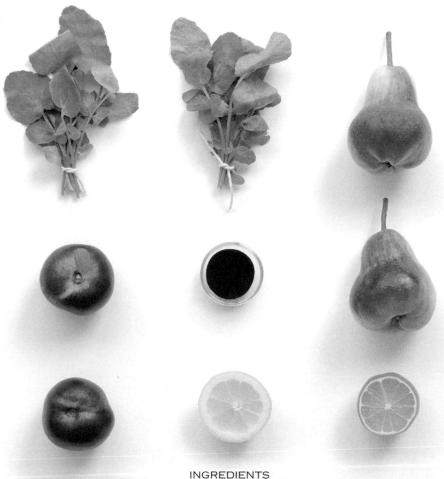

INGREDIENTS
2 handfuls of watercress

½ lime • ½ lemon

2 pears • 2 nectarines • 1 teaspoon spirulina

Juice all the ingredients apart from the spirulina. Put the spirulina in a glass, then stir in the juice slowly so the powder combines well into the juice. Spirulina is found in most health food shops, and it's also available online.

This juice is not only great for your brain, but contains a high quantity of vitamin B-12, which is essential for healthy nerves and tissues.

MB *Metabolism boosting* **A** *Alkalising* **AO** *Anti-oxidising*

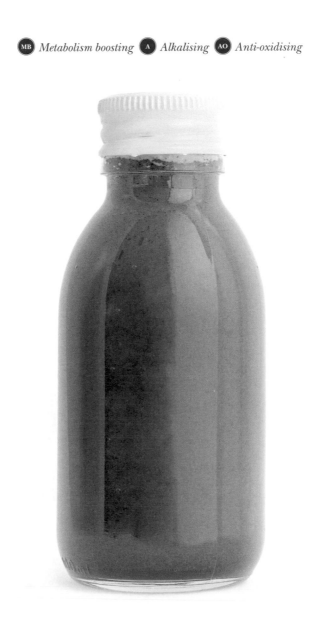

POPEYE'S JUICE
Slightly sweet

INGREDIENTS
2 handfuls of spinach
⅓ pineapple
2 handfuls of raspberries

Juice all the ingredients

This juice is high in vitamins and minerals and will give you a fantastic iron boost.

MB *Metabolism boosting* **SE** *Skin enhancing* **DE** *Digestion enhancing*

FAT BURNER

Savoury

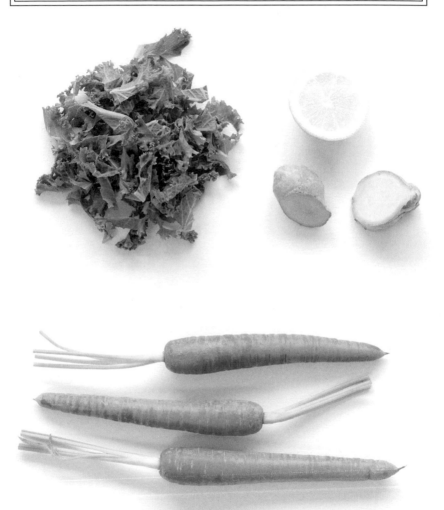

INGREDIENTS

3 carrots

A handful of kale

½ lemon • 2 thumbs of ginger

Juice all the ingredients.

This stimulating juice, which is rich in fibre, gets the blood pumping round your body, fighting off any infections in its way.

MB *Metabolism boosting* **MBB** *Muscle & bone building* **I** *Immunising*

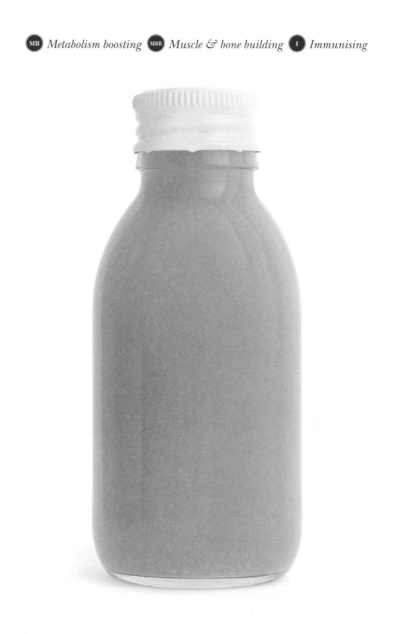

DIGESTIVO

Earthy

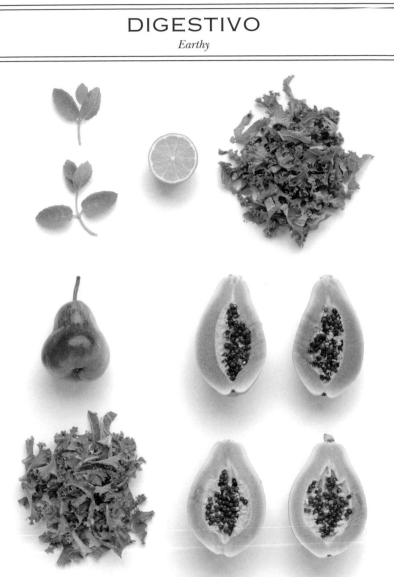

INGREDIENTS
2 papayas • 2 handfuls of kale
1 pear • 2 sprigs of mint
½ lime

Juice all the ingredients.

This juice helps to replenish your vitamin C and
also has a calming effect on the body.

BN *Blood nourishing* **DE** *Digestion enhancing* **AI** *Anti-inflammatory*

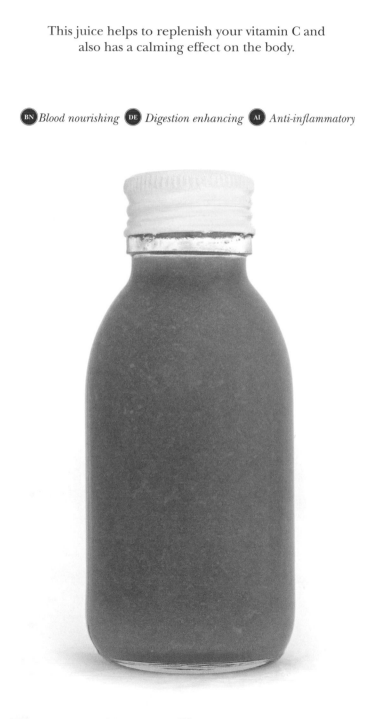

FULL OF TOMATOES
Savoury

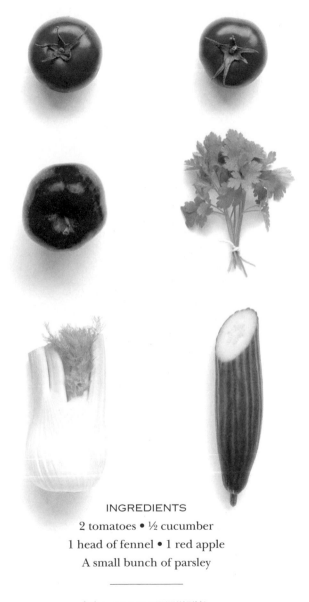

INGREDIENTS
2 tomatoes • ½ cucumber
1 head of fennel • 1 red apple
A small bunch of parsley

Juice all the ingredients.

This juice contains lots of lycopene, which is great for your heart.

SE *Skin enhancing* De *Detoxifying* I *Immunising*

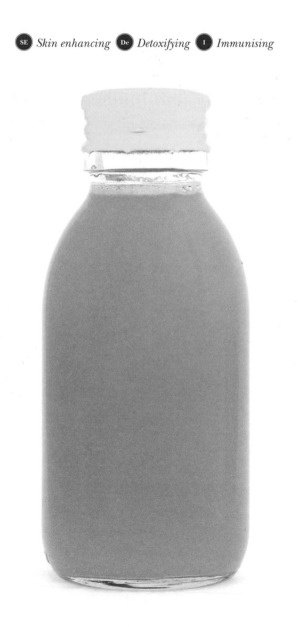

BERRY INFECTIOUS
Sweet

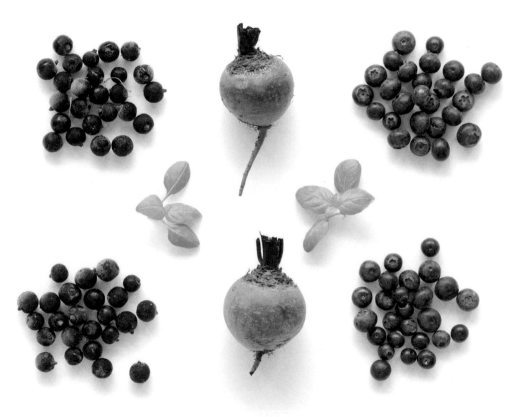

INGREDIENTS
2 handfuls of blueberries

2 handfuls of blackcurrants

2 sprigs of basil • 2 beetroots

Juice all the ingredients.

Packed with antioxidants, this juice is great for your blood.

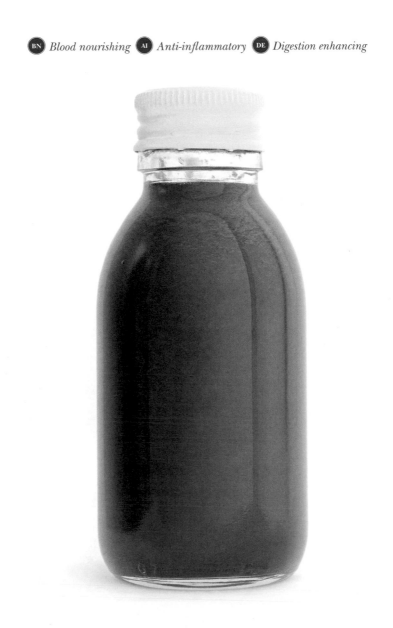 *Blood nourishing* 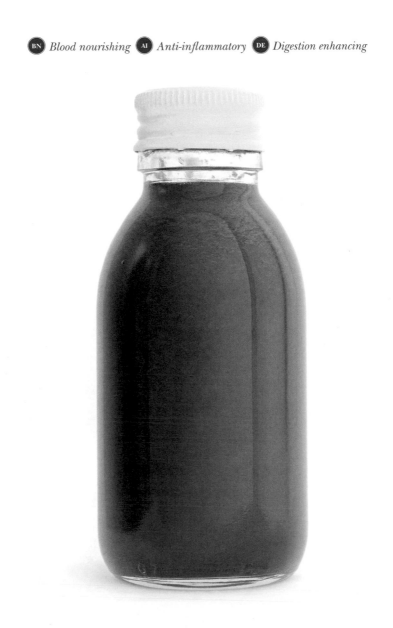 *Anti-inflammatory* 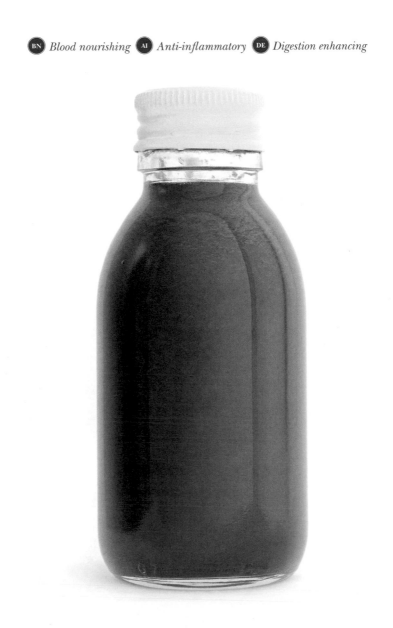 *Digestion enhancing*

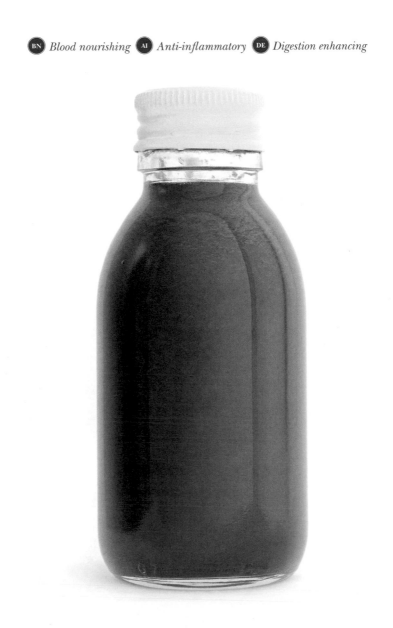

RASPBERRY MINT
Sweet

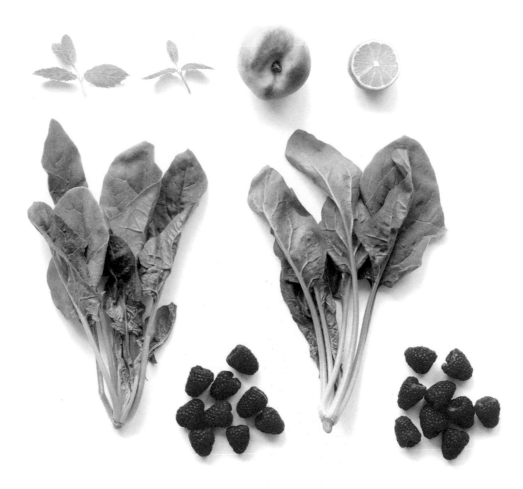

INGREDIENTS
2 handfuls of raspberries • ½ lime
2 sprigs of mint • 1 peach
2 handfuls of spinach

Juice all the ingredients

High in vitamin C and antioxidants, this juice
is great for overall health.

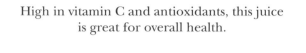

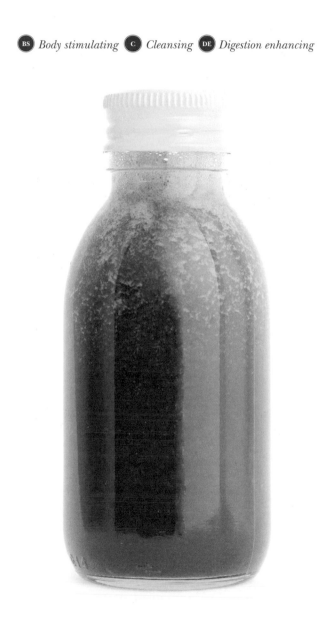

STRAWBERRY

A little sweet

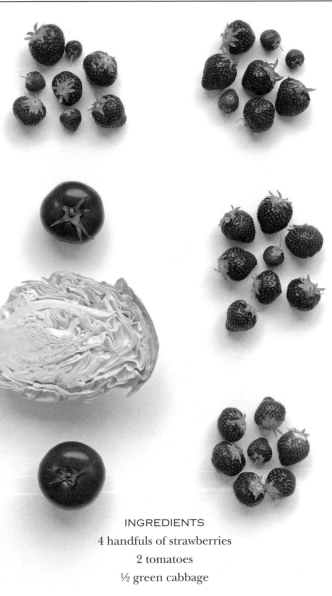

INGREDIENTS

4 handfuls of strawberries

2 tomatoes

½ green cabbage

Juice all the ingredients.

This juice helps to boost your cardiovascular system and is an excellent source of vitamin C.

FF *Fat flushing* **BN** *Blood nourishing* **I** *Immunising*

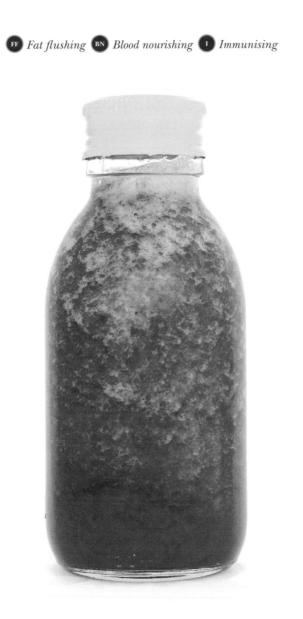

DETOXIFIER

A little sweet

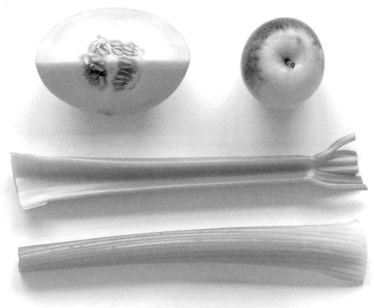

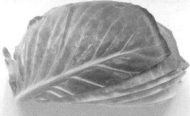

INGREDIENTS
¼ green cabbage • 1 apple
2 sticks of celery
¼ Galia melon

Juice all the ingredients.

This juice is a great cleanser for your liver and is rich in vitamins C and K.

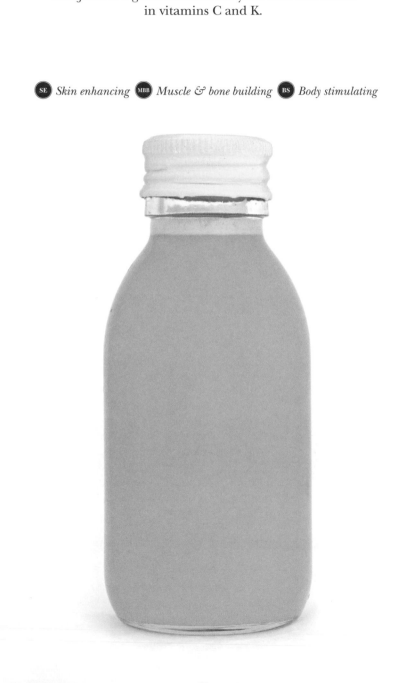

SE *Skin enhancing* **MBB** *Muscle & bone building* **BS** *Body stimulating*

FULL OF CARROTS

A little sweet

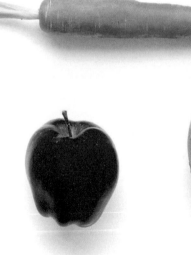

INGREDIENTS

4 carrots

1 red apple

1 sweet potato

Juice all the ingredients.

A boost for all your organs as well as your skin, this juice is rich in beta-carotene and vitamin A.

I *Immunising* **BP** *Brain powering* **SE** *Skin enhancing*

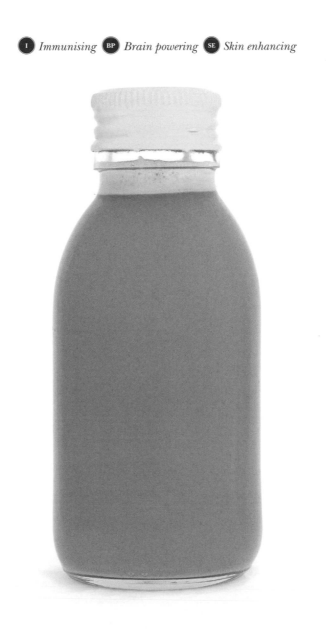

THE CLEANSER
Savoury

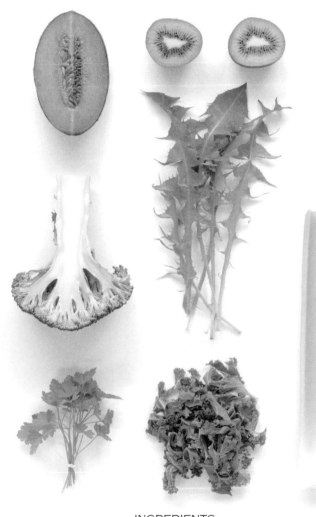

INGREDIENTS
A stick of celery • A small bunch of parsley
A handful of kale • ½ small head of broccoli
A small bunch of dandelion greens • ¼ cantaloupe melon • 1 kiwi

Juice all the ingredients

High in potassium and calcium, this is one of the
best juices you can make.

SE *Skin enhancing* **DE** *Digestion enhancing* **BS** *Body stimulating*

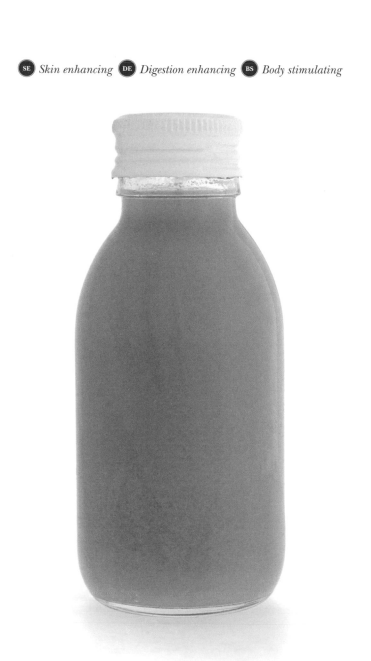

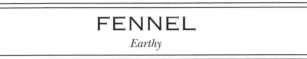

FENNEL
Earthy

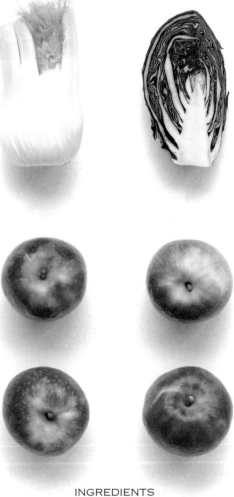

INGREDIENTS
1 head of fennel
¼ red cabbage
4 red apples

Juice all the ingredients.

This juice is rich in vitamin C and also helps to reduce inflammation.

De *Detoxifying* **BN** *Blood nourishing* **DE** *Digestion enhancing*

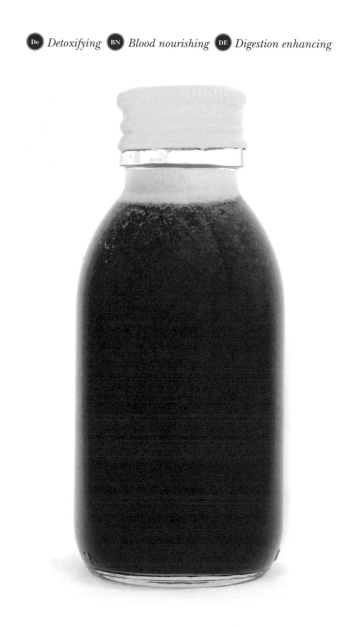

PURPLE GINGER
Sweet

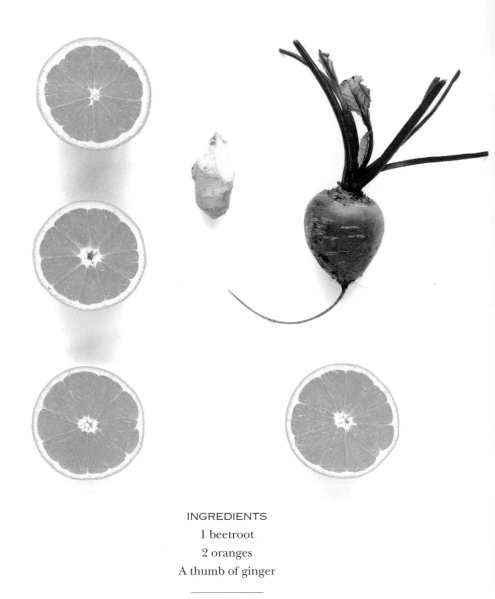

INGREDIENTS

1 beetroot

2 oranges

A thumb of ginger

Juice all the ingredients.

A great juice to drink before you exercise, this helps the
uptake of oxygen in blood cells.

MB *Metabolism boosting*   **BS** *Body stimulating*   **BN** *Blood nourishing*

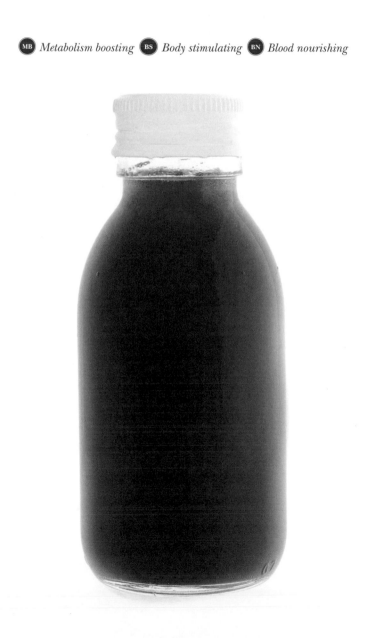

SMOOTHIES

Smoothies are really simple to make. You can produce them in vast quantities and keep them in the refrigerator for a few days. Most of these smoothies make 500ml with 100–200ml of water added. You can add as much water as you like to achieve your preferred consistency. Some smoothies are thicker than others, so you will have to add more or less depending on the ingredients. When lemons, oranges and limes are listed in the ingredients, just peel them and then blend the whole fruit. Sometimes, the recipe will specify that you should juice them first to give more liquid.

STRAWBERRY JOY

Sweet

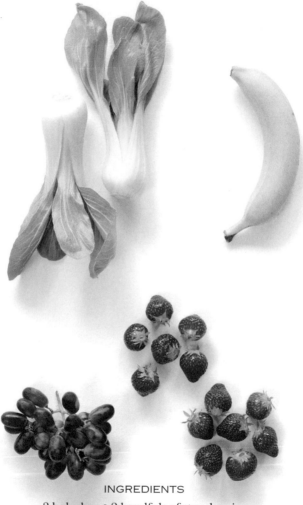

INGREDIENTS

2 bok choy • 2 handfuls of strawberries

A small bunch of red grapes

1 banana

Blend the ingredients. Add more water, if necessary, to reach
your desired consistency, then drink.

This smoothie contains lots of vitamin K, which helps to build strong bones and reduce inflammation.

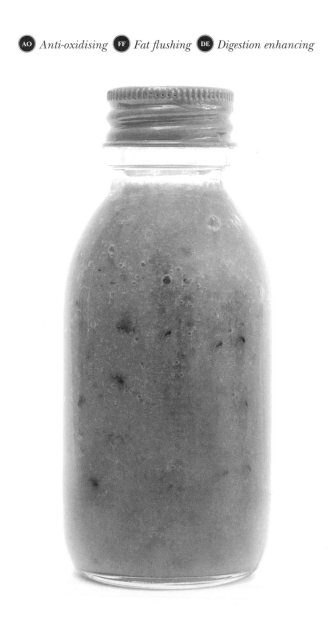 AO *Anti-oxidising* FF *Fat flushing* DE *Digestion enhancing*

SMOOTH SPINACH BERRY

Sweet

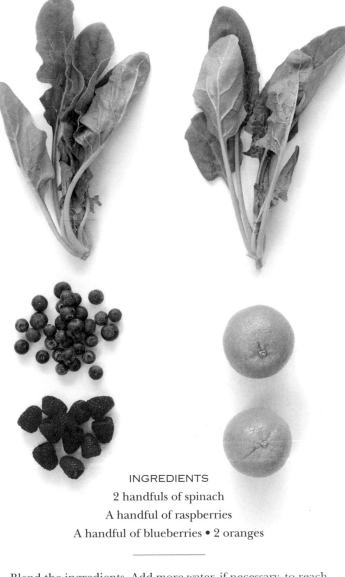

INGREDIENTS

2 handfuls of spinach

A handful of raspberries

A handful of blueberries • 2 oranges

Blend the ingredients. Add more water, if necessary, to reach your desired consistency, then drink.

A smoothie full of vitamins and lots of iron, which helps
to fight urinary infections.

BN *Blood nourishing* SE *Skin enhancing* C *Cleansing*

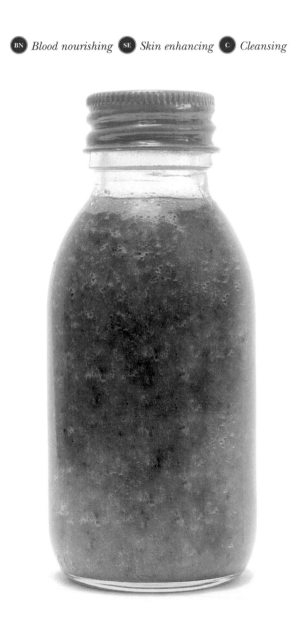

BANANA TONIC

Slightly sweet

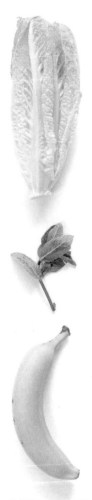

INGREDIENTS

1 romaine lettuce

1 banana

A sprig of mint

Blend the ingredients. Add more water, if necessary, to reach
your desired consistency, then drink.

This smoothie helps to give your body a sense of calm and is a good source of vitamin B-6, vitamin C and potassium.

D *Diuretic* **BN** *Blood nourishing* **AI** *Anti-inflammatory*

TROPICAL CABBAGE
Sweet

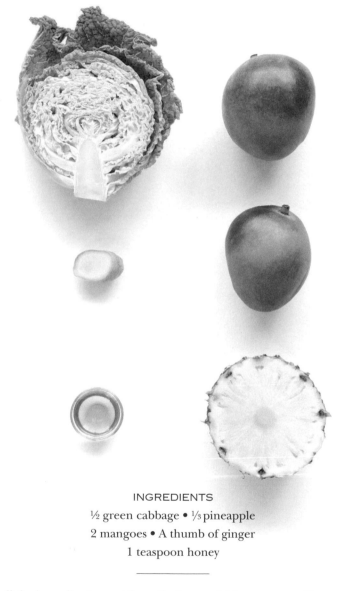

INGREDIENTS
½ green cabbage • ⅓ pineapple

2 mangoes • A thumb of ginger

1 teaspoon honey

Blend all the ingredients apart from the honey. Add more water if necessary to reach your desired consistency. Stir in the honey, then drink.

Rich in vitamins C and K, this smoothie also aids digestion.

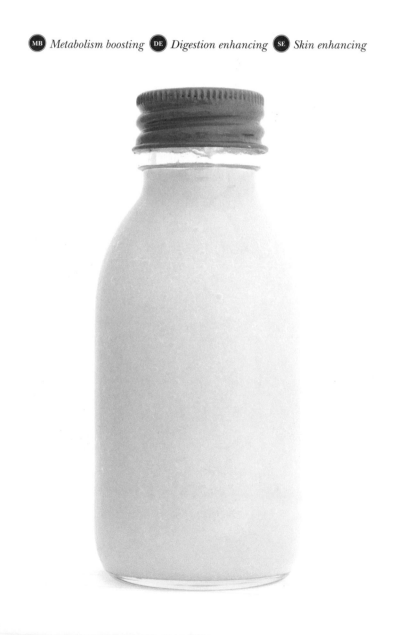

MB *Metabolism boosting* **DE** *Digestion enhancing* **SE** *Skin enhancing*

COCONUT KALE

Sweet

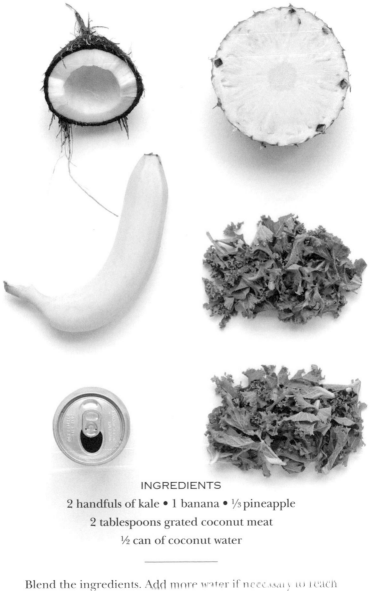

INGREDIENTS

2 handfuls of kale • 1 banana • ⅓ pineapple

2 tablespoons grated coconut meat

½ can of coconut water

Blend the ingredients. Add more water if necessary to reach
your desired consistency, then drink.

Rich in vitamins A, C and K, this is a great anti-bacterial smoothie.

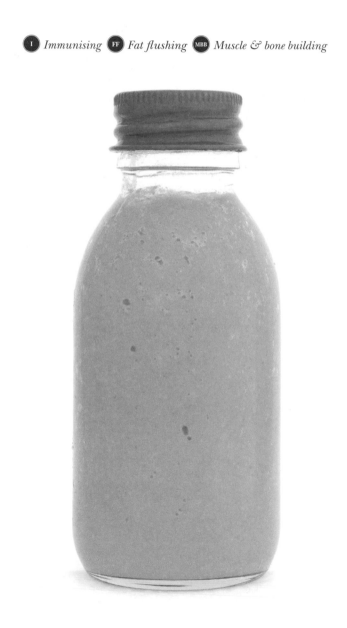 *Immunising* 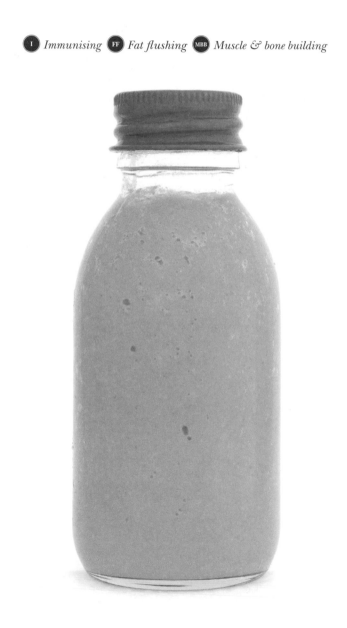 *Fat flushing* 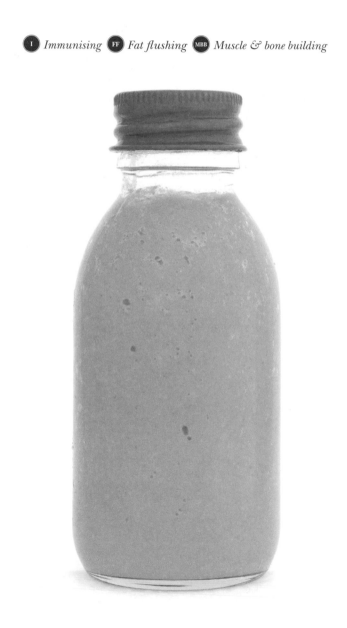 *Muscle & bone building*

HEARTY PEAR

Slightly sweet

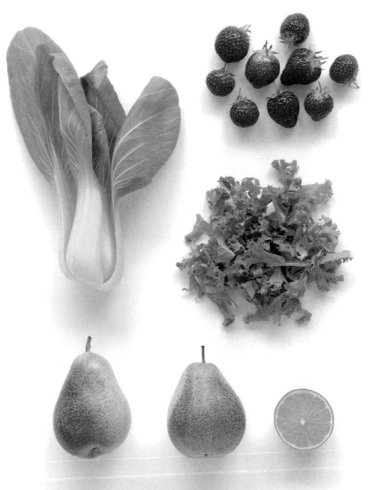

INGREDIENTS
A handful of kale • 1 bok choy

2 pears • A handful of strawberries

A squeeze of lime

Blend the ingredients. Add more water if necessary to
reach your desired consistency, then drink.

High in antioxidants, this smoothie is also great for your eyes.

DE *Digestion enhancing* **I** *Immunising* **BN** *Blood nourishing*

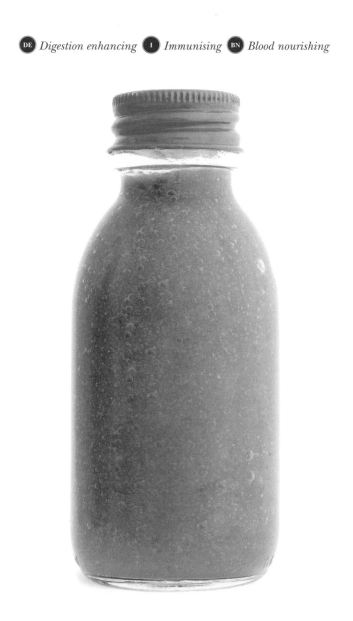

HIGH ON FIBRE

Slightly sweet

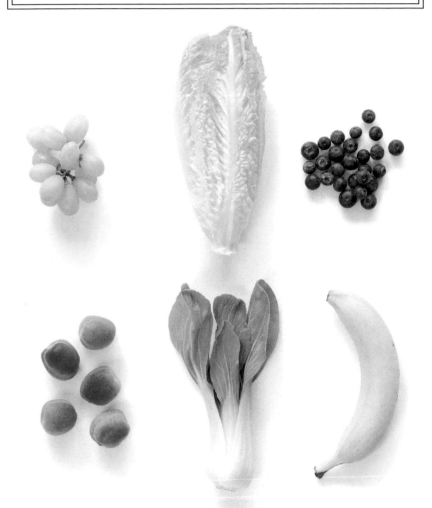

INGREDIENTS

1 romaine lettuce • 1 bok choy

5 apricots • A handful of blueberries

1 banana • A small bunch of green grapes

Blend the ingredients. Add more water, if necessary, to reach
your desired consistency, then drink.

Rich in vitamins C and K, this smoothie is great for
your digestive system.

C *Cleansing* **BN** *Blood nourishing* **De** *Detoxifying*

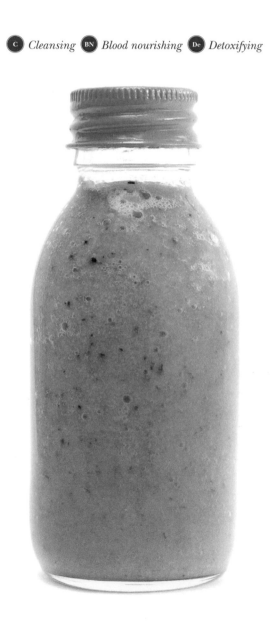

ALKALINER

Slightly sweet

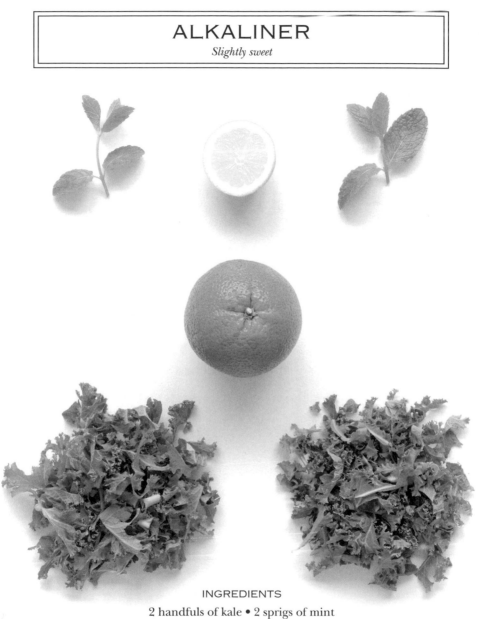

INGREDIENTS

2 handfuls of kale • 2 sprigs of mint
1 orange • ½ lemon

Blend the ingredients. Add more water, if necessary, to reach
your desired consistency, then drink.

This smoothie is known to be a good stress reliever and is rich in vitamins A, C and K.

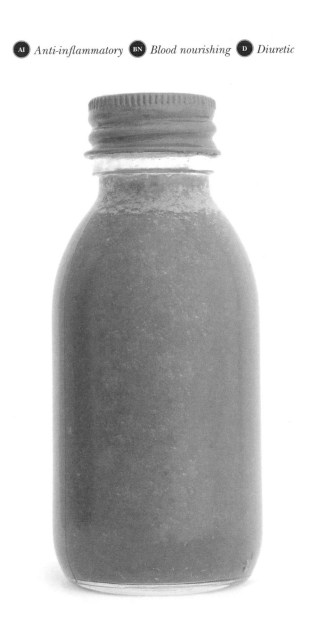 Anti-inflammatory 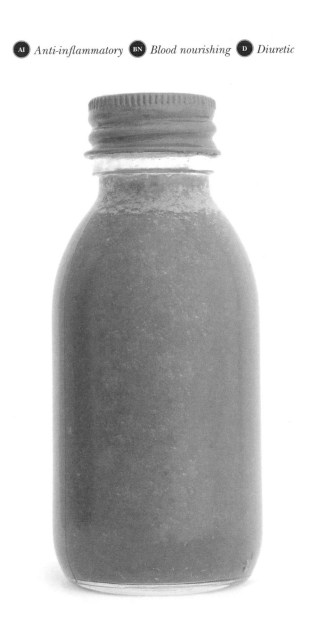 Blood nourishing 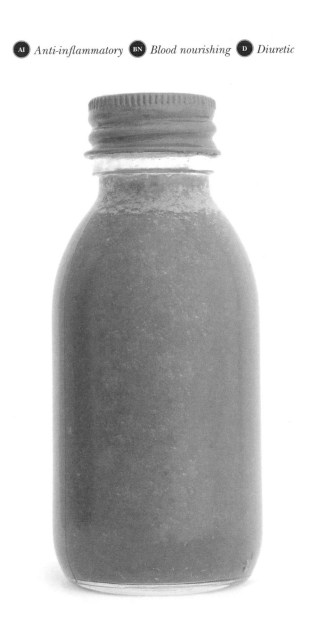 Diuretic

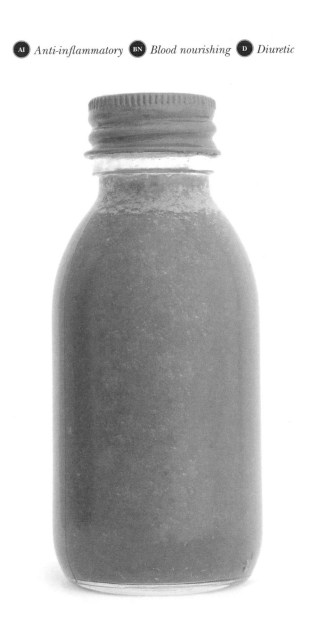

BLUEBERRY KALE

Slightly sweet

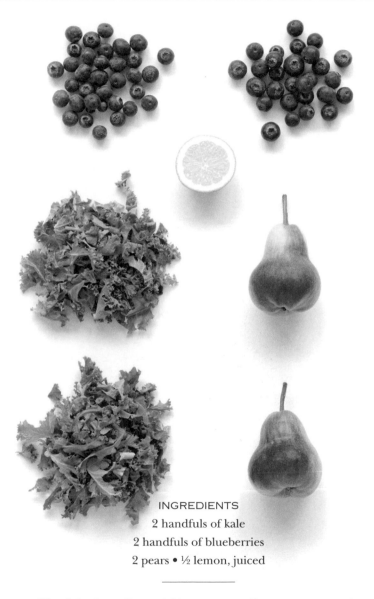

INGREDIENTS
2 handfuls of kale

2 handfuls of blueberries

2 pears • ½ lemon, juiced

Blend the ingredients. Add more water, if necessary, to reach
your desired consistency, then drink.

Full of vitamins A, C and K, this smoothie is good
for enriching your blood.

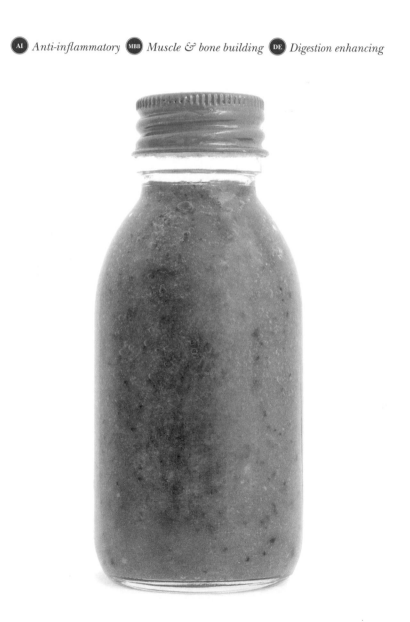 *Anti-inflammatory* 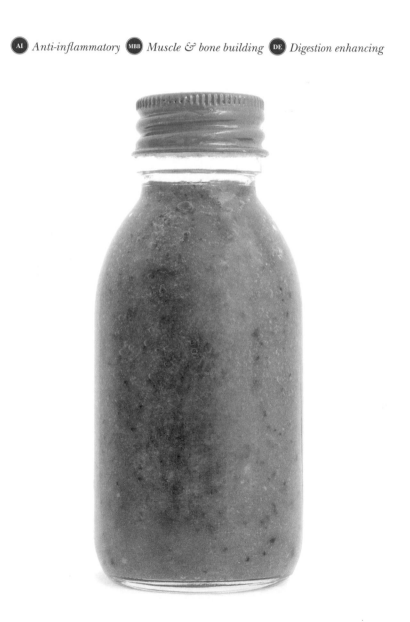 *Muscle & bone building* 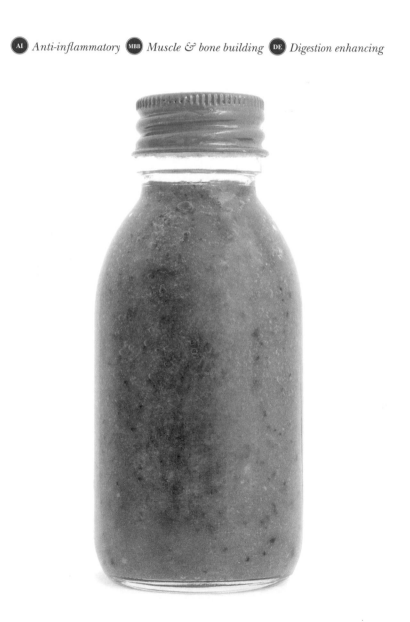 *Digestion enhancing*

PEACHY

Slightly sweet

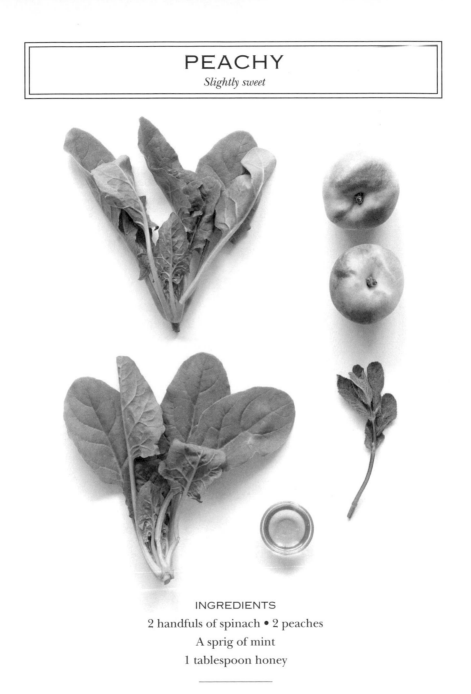

INGREDIENTS

2 handfuls of spinach • 2 peaches

A sprig of mint

1 tablespoon honey

Blend the ingredients apart from the honey. Add more water if necessary to reach your desired consistency, top with honey and then drink.

Peaches are great at helping you feel full as well as being packed with vitamin C, vitamin A and potassium.

BS *Body stimulating* **BN** *Blood nourishing* **MBB** *Muscle & bone building*

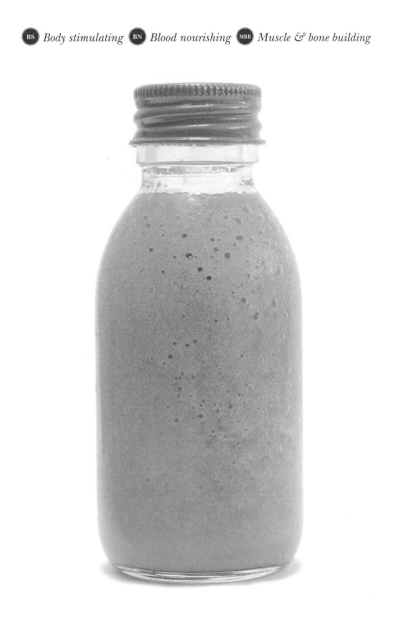

AVOCADO
Slightly savoury

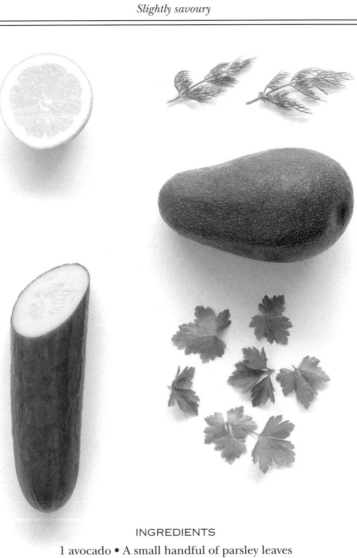

INGREDIENTS
1 avocado • A small handful of parsley leaves
½ cucumber • 2 sprigs of dill
½ lemon, juiced

Blend the ingredients. Add more water, if necessary, to reach
your desired consistency, then drink.

This smoothie, which is high in chlorophyll, is
great at cleansing your vital organs.

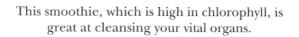 *Blood nourishing* *Anti-inflammatory* *Cleansing*

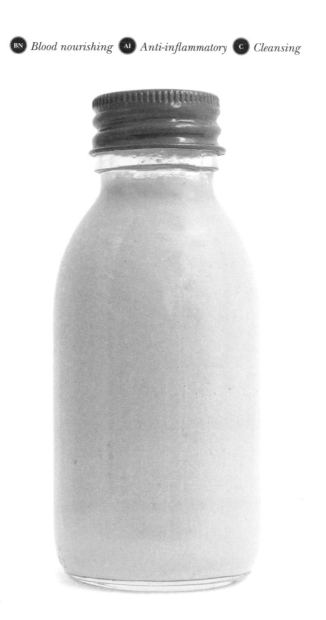

TOMATO & BASIL

Savoury

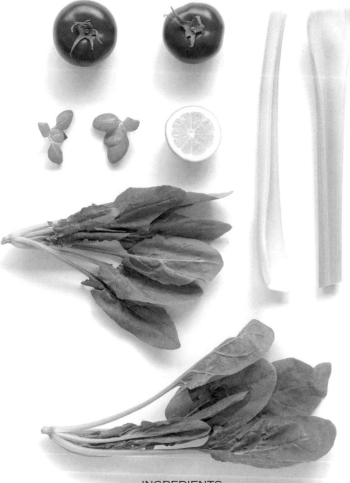

INGREDIENTS

2 tomatoes • 2 sprigs of basil

2 sticks of celery • 2 handfuls of spinach

A squeeze of lemon

Blend the ingredients. Add more water, if necessary, to
reach your desired consistency, then drink.

Tomatoes are known to help lower your risk of cancer because they are full of antioxidants.

SE *Skin enhancing* **C** *Cleansing* **BS** *Body stimulating*

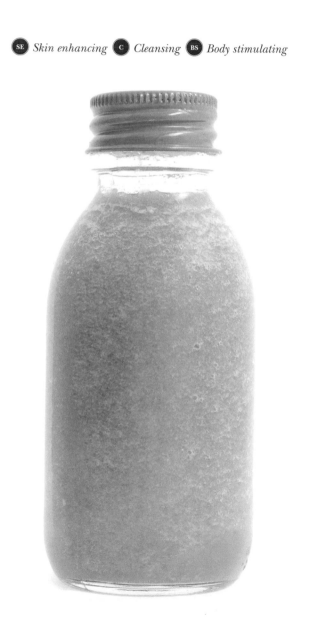

CORIANDER PEPPER

Savoury

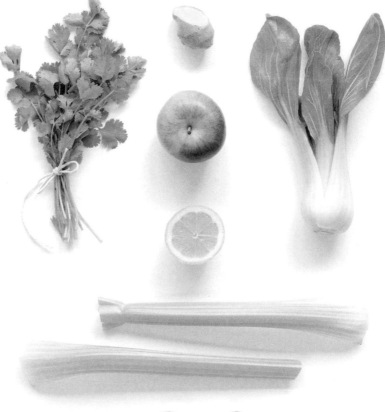

INGREDIENTS

A handful of coriander leaves • 1 bok choy • 1 apple
2 sticks of celery • A thumb of ginger • A pinch of turmeric
A pinch of cayenne pepper • A squeeze of lemon

Blend the ingredients. Add more water, if necessary, to
reach your desired consistency, then drink.

This smoothie is high in iron and is great at combating various digestive ailments.

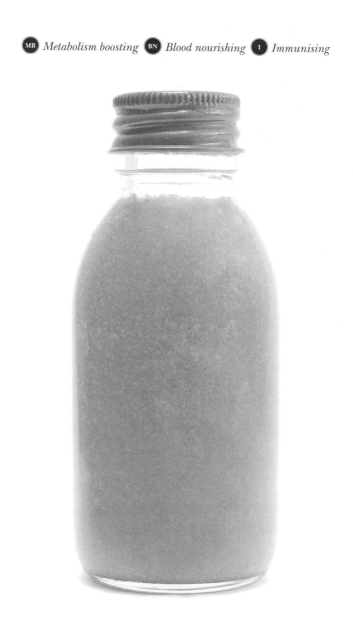

MB *Metabolism boosting* **BN** *Blood nourishing* **I** *Immunising*

Savoury spice

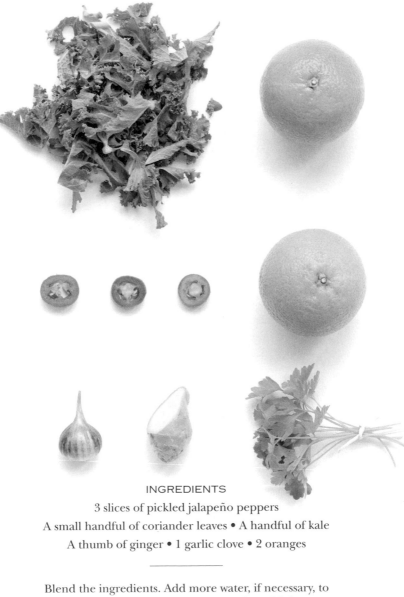

INGREDIENTS
3 slices of pickled jalapeño peppers

A small handful of coriander leaves • A handful of kale

A thumb of ginger • 1 garlic clove • 2 oranges

Blend the ingredients. Add more water, if necessary, to
reach your desired consistency, then drink.

This smoothie has great healing properties and
is also high in vitamins A, C and K.

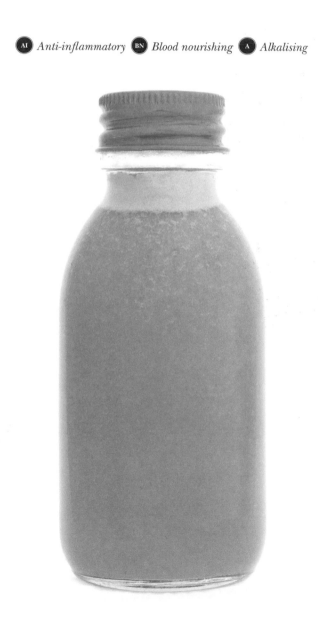

AI *Anti-inflammatory* *BN* *Blood nourishing* *A* *Alkalising*

FENNEL BREEZE

Savoury

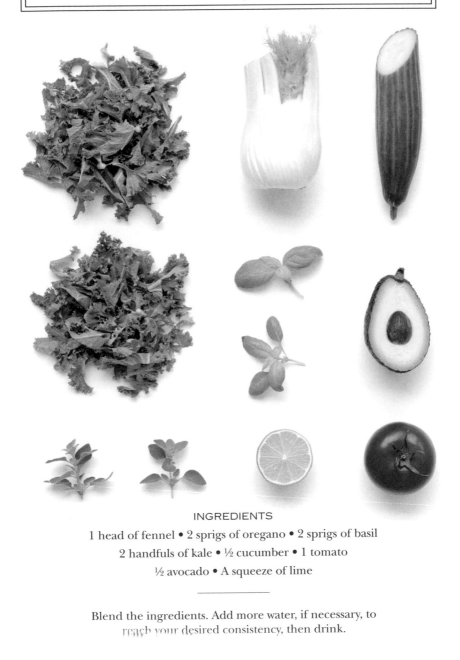

INGREDIENTS

1 head of fennel • 2 sprigs of oregano • 2 sprigs of basil
2 handfuls of kale • ½ cucumber • 1 tomato
½ avocado • A squeeze of lime

Blend the ingredients. Add more water, if necessary, to
reach your desired consistency, then drink.

Treat your skin by drinking this smoothie, which is rich in vitamin C and fibre.

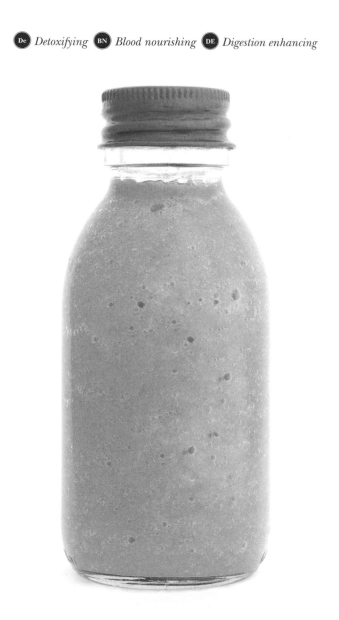 **De** *Detoxifying* **BN** *Blood nourishing* **DE** *Digestion enhancing*

KICKSTART YOUR MORNING
Savoury

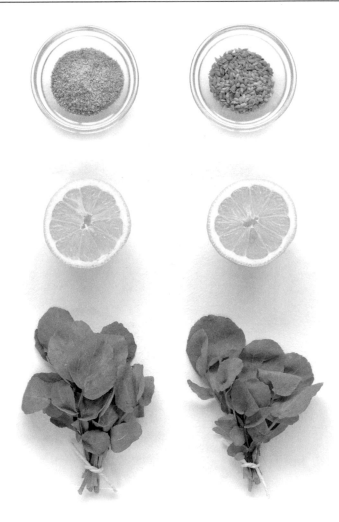

INGREDIENTS
2 handfuls of watercress • 1 tablespoon wheatgerm
1 tablespoon linseed • 1 lemon, juiced

Blend the ingredients. Add more water, if necessary, to reach your desired
consistency, then drink. Add honey if you like a little sweetness.

This body-boosting smoothie brightens up every cell in your body and is rich in vitamin A, vitamin K and calcium.

BS *Body stimulating* **BN** *Blood nourishing* **FF** *Fat flushing*

FRUITY FERTILITY

Slightly sweet

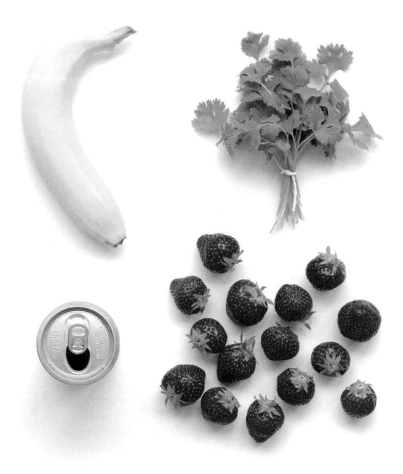

INGREDIENTS

A big bunch of coriander leaves

2 handfuls of strawberries

½ can of coconut water • 1 banana

Blend the ingredients. Add more water, if necessary, to
reach your desired consistency, then drink.

This smoothie helps to reduce cholesterol and is rich in fibre.

De *Detoxifying* **FF** *Fat flushing* **BS** *Body stimulating*

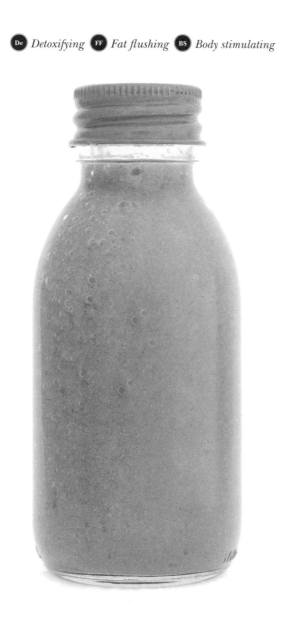

VANILLA & FIGS

Slightly sweet

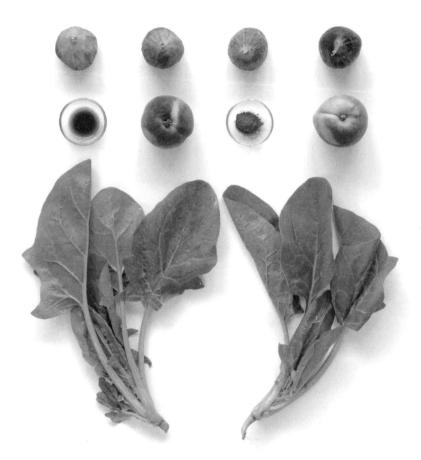

INGREDIENTS

4 small figs or 2 large ones • 2 handfuls of spinach

2 peaches • A pinch of cinnamon

2 drops of vanilla extract

Blend the ingredients. Add more water, if necessary, to
reach your desired consistency, then drink.

Rich in fibre and potassium, this is a great calming smoothie for those who suffer from anxiety.

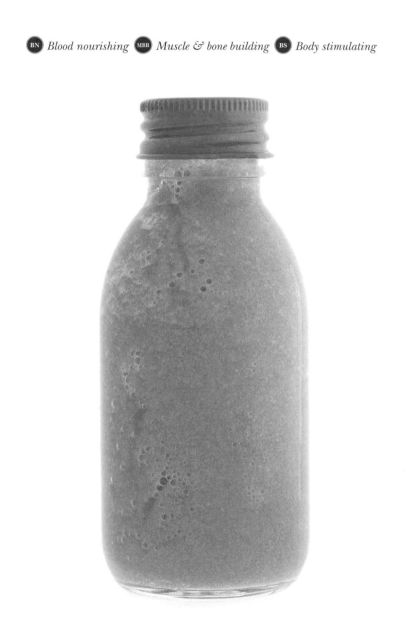 **BN** *Blood nourishing* **MBB** *Muscle & bone building* **BS** *Body stimulating*

PINEAPPLE TWIST

Slightly sweet

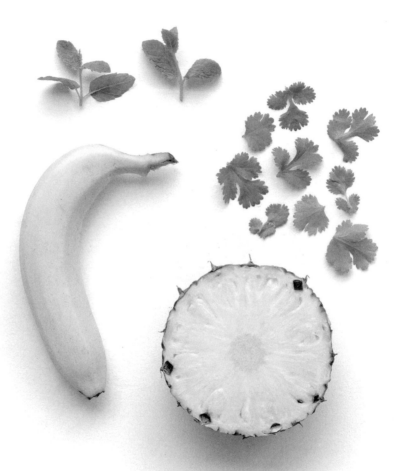

INGREDIENTS

⅓ pineapple

A small handful of coriander leaves

1 banana • 2 sprigs of mint

Blend the ingredients. Add more water, if necessary, to
reach your desired consistency, then drink.

Rich in vitamin C, this smoothie helps to aid your digestion.

DE *Digestion enhancing* **AI** *Anti-inflammatory* **De** *Detoxifying*

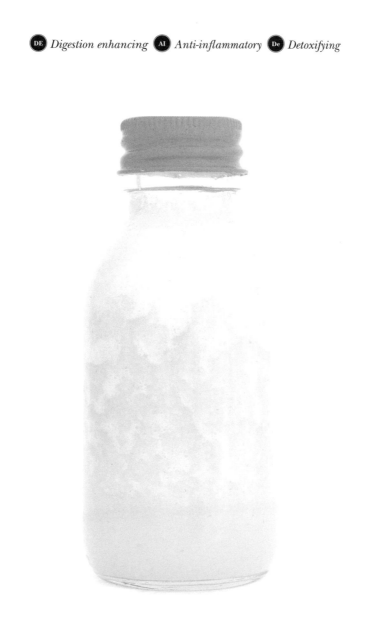

NECTARINE SOUR
Bitter sweet

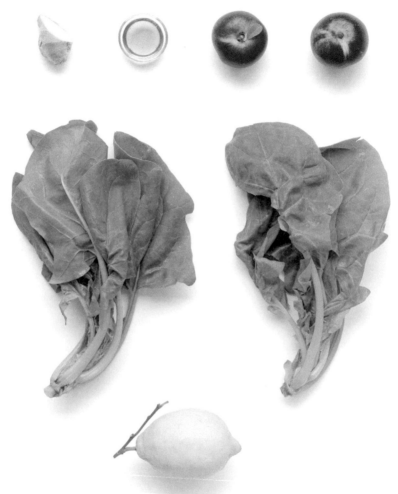

INGREDIENTS
2 handfuls of spinach • 2 nectarines
A thumb of ginger • 1 tablespoon honey
1 lemon, whole including peel and pith

Blend the ingredients. Add more water, if necessary, to reach your desired
consistency, then drink.

This smoothie helps to prevent allergies and is full of vitamins and iron.

Di *Diuretic* A *Alkalising* AI *Anti-inflammatory*

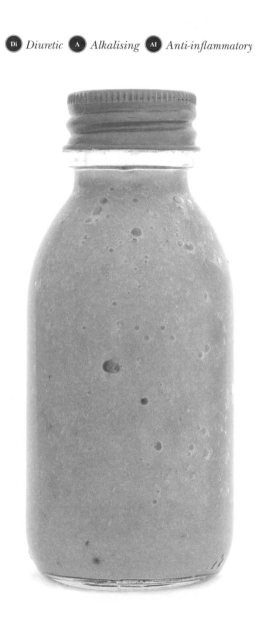

KING OF THE FRUITS

Slightly sweet

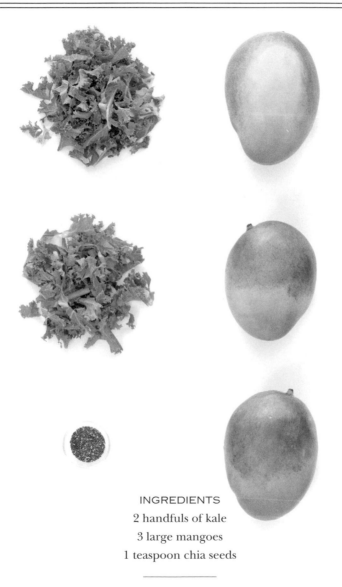

INGREDIENTS
2 handfuls of kale
3 large mangoes
1 teaspoon chia seeds

Blend all the ingredients. The chia seeds thicken this smoothie, so add enough water to reach your desired consistency. Chia seeds can be bought from most health food shops and are available online.

This smoothie will give you a big boost of vitamins A, C and K.

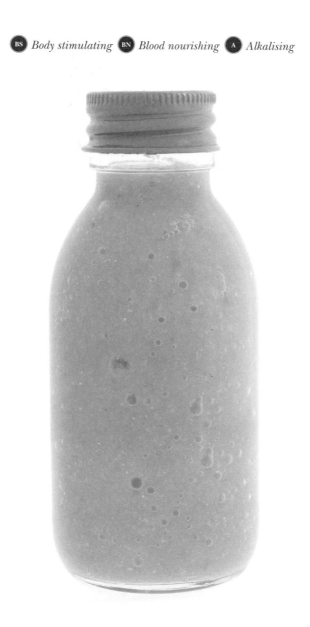 *Body stimulating* 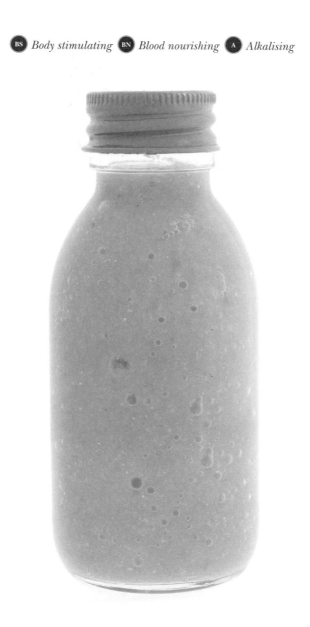 *Blood nourishing* 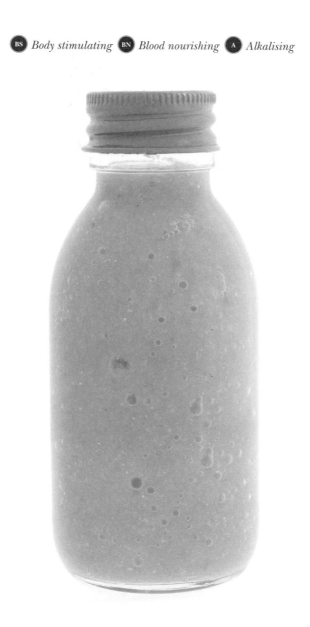 *Alkalising*

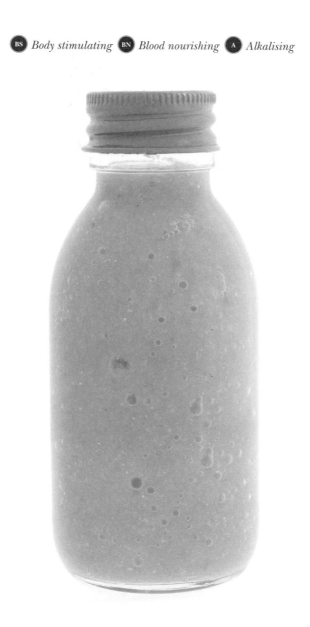

WATERMELON

Slightly sweet

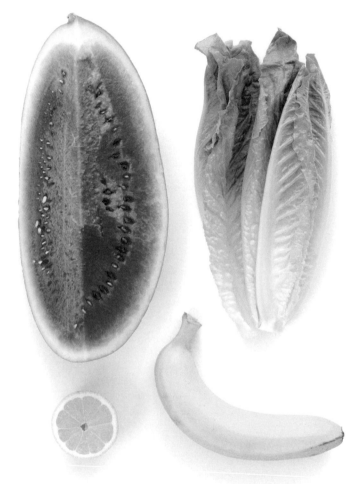

INGREDIENTS

¾ small watermelon or ¼ large watermelon, seeds removed

1 romaine lettuce • 1 banana

A squeeze of lemon

Blend the ingredients apart from the lemon. Add more water, if necessary, to reach your desired consistency. Add a squeeze of lemon, then drink.

114

Rich in lycopene, this smoothie is great for flushing out your kidneys and bladder.

AO *Anti-oxidising* **I** *Immunising* **Di** *Diuretic*

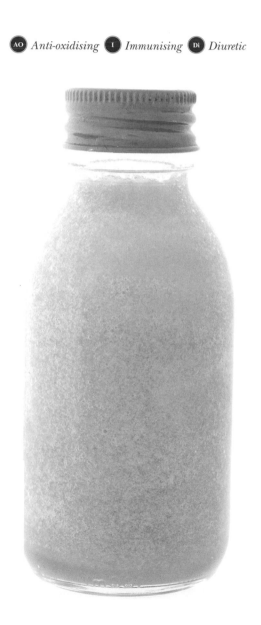

GREEN PAPAYA

Slightly sweet

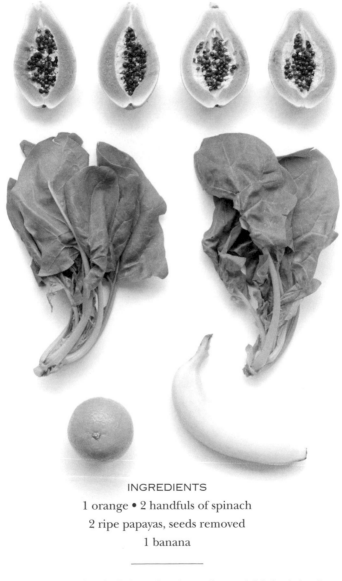

INGREDIENTS

1 orange • 2 handfuls of spinach

2 ripe papayas, seeds removed

1 banana

Juice the orange first. Blend all the other ingredients. Add the juiced orange to the smoothie. Add water until it reaches your desired consistency, then drink.

Rich in vitamin C and iron, this juice also
helps your body fight cancer.

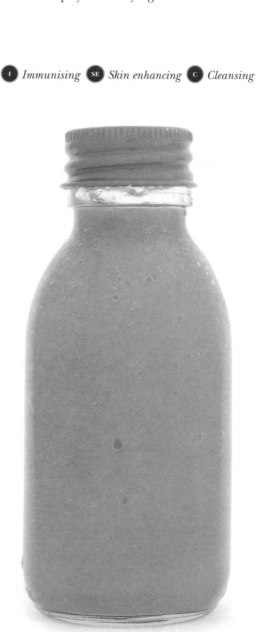 Immunising SE Skin enhancing C Cleansing

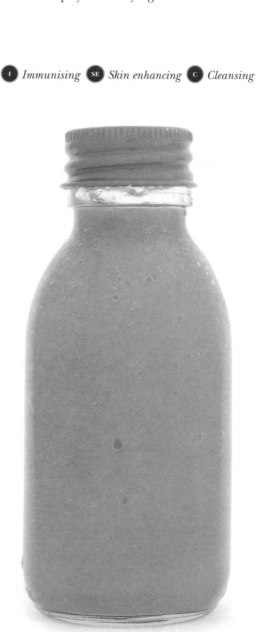

SUPER CANTALOUPE

Slightly sweet

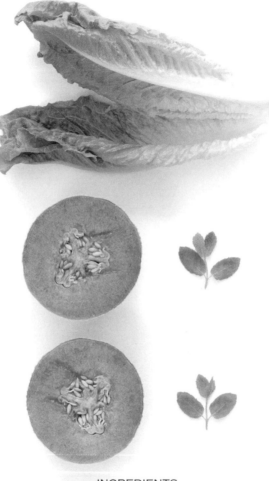

INGREDIENTS

1 romaine lettuce

1 cantaloupe melon

2 sprigs of mint

Blend the ingredients. Add more water, if necessary, to
reach your desired consistency, then drink.

Rich in vitamins A and K, this smoothie is a powerful cleanser, which also helps with anxiety.

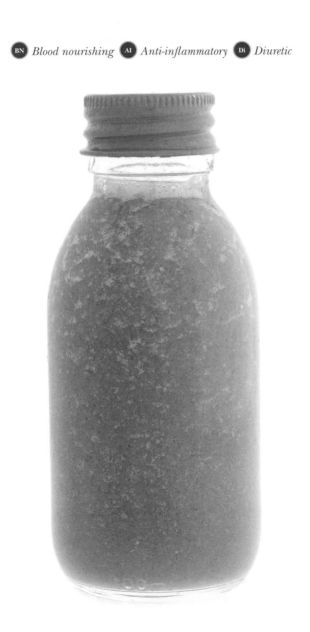 Blood nourishing 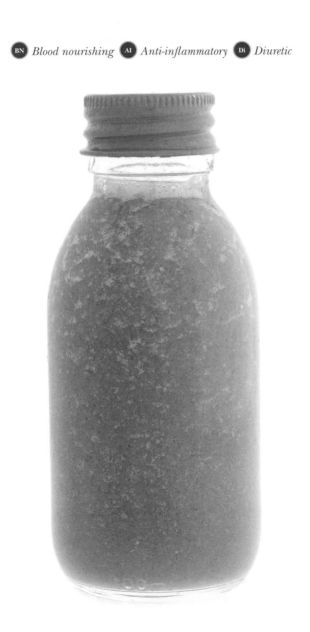 Anti-inflammatory 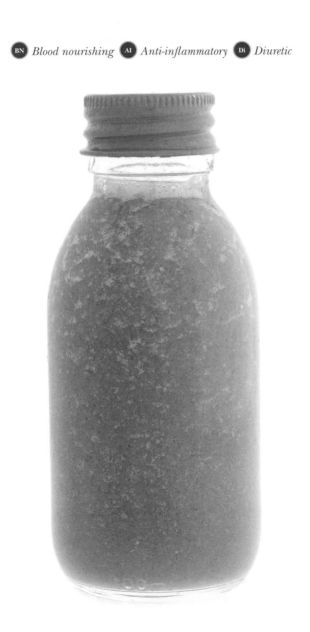 Diuretic

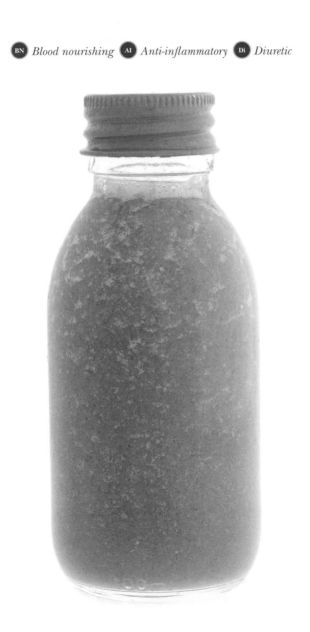

BLACKCURRANTS

Sweet

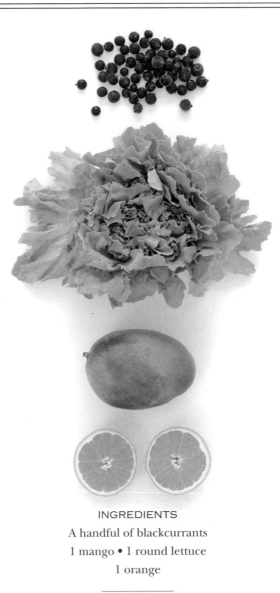

INGREDIENTS

A handful of blackcurrants

1 mango • 1 round lettuce

1 orange

Blend the ingredients. Add more water, if necessary, to reach your desired
consistency, then drink.

Packed with vitamin A, vitamin B-6 and potassium, this smoothie can also help with urinary infections.

Immunising _Body stimulating_ _Brain powering_

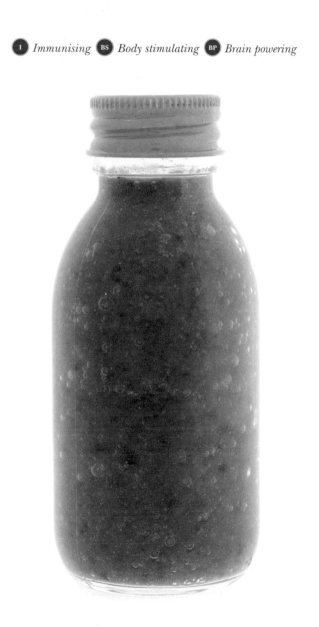

ALOE LEAF

Slightly sweet

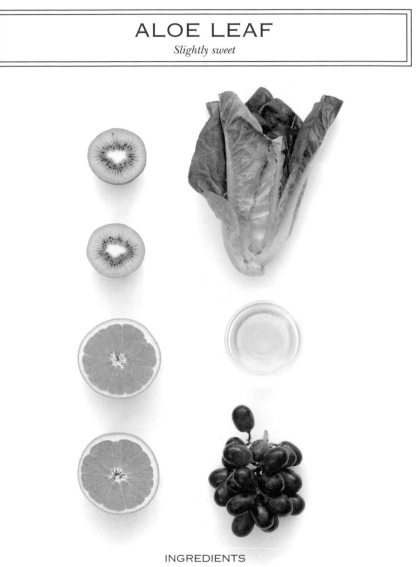

INGREDIENTS

1 tablespoon aloe vera juice

A small bunch of red grapes

1 red leaf lettuce • 1 kiwi • 1 orange

Blend the ingredients. Add more water, if necessary, to reach
your desired consistency, then drink. Aloe vera juice can be
found in most health food shops or online.

High in vitamin C, this smoothie also helps
improve your blood circulation.

SE *Skin enhancing* **De** *Detoxifying* **DE** *Digestion enhancing*

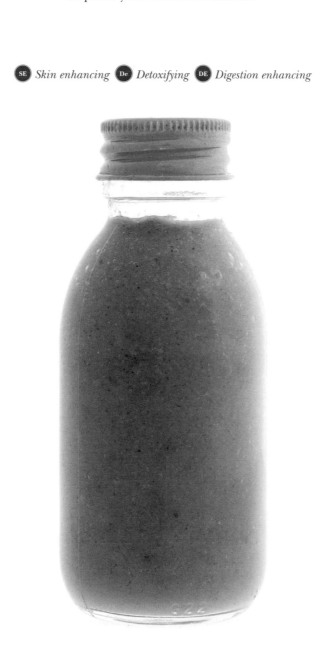

GOJI TANGERINE

Slightly sweet

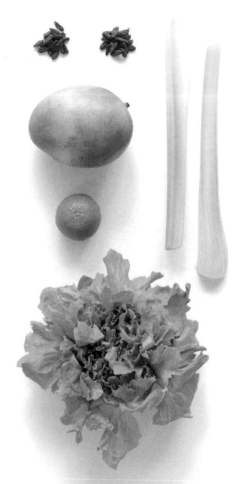

INGREDIENTS

2 teaspoons dried goji berries

1 mango • 1 tangerine

2 sticks of celery • 1 round lettuce

Blend the ingredients. Add more water, if necessary, to reach your desired
consistency, and drink. Goji berries can be found in most supermarkets,
health food shops or online.

This smoothie is packed with vitamin C and beta-carotene, which enhance your skin and reduce inflammation.

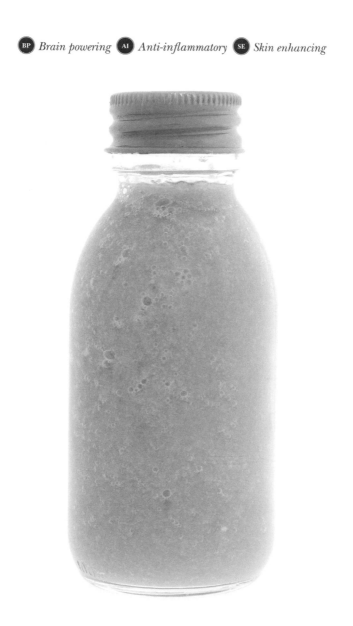 **BP** *Brain powering* **AI** *Anti-inflammatory* **SE** *Skin enhancing*

EASTERN JUICE

Slightly sweet

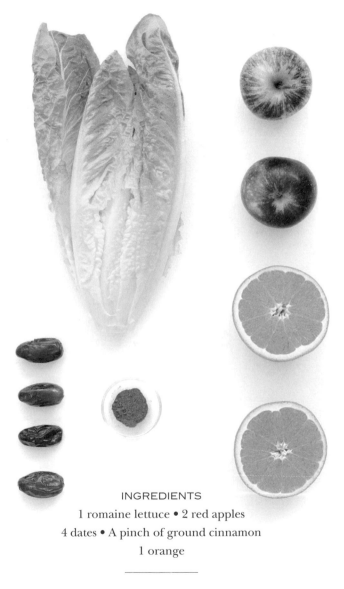

INGREDIENTS

1 romaine lettuce • 2 red apples
4 dates • A pinch of ground cinnamon
1 orange

Blend the ingredients. Add more water, if necessary, to
reach your desired consistency, then drink.

This smoothie helps lower your cholesterol as well as being full of vitamins A, C and K.

BN *Blood nourishing* **FF** *Fat flushing* **DE** *Digestion enhancing*

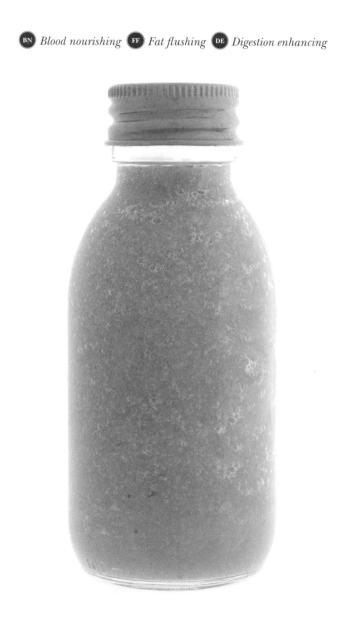

LEEK & CUCUMBER

Savoury

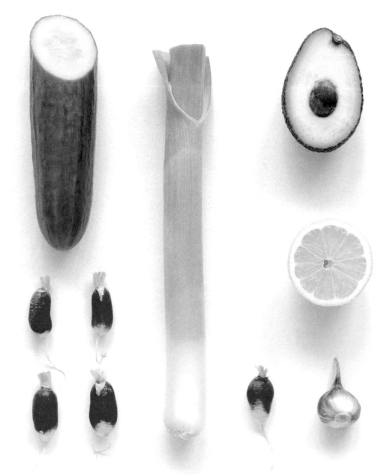

INGREDIENTS

1 leek • ½ cucumber

½ avocado • 5 radishes

1 garlic clove • ½ lemon

Blend the ingredients. Add more water, if necessary, to
reach your desired consistency, then drink. If you fancy a bit
of spice, add a few slices of jalapeño pepper.

Rich in kaempferol and folate, this smoothie helps to cleanse your body from the build-up of toxins.

SE *Skin enhancing* **DE** *Digestion enhancing* **BS** *Body stimulating*

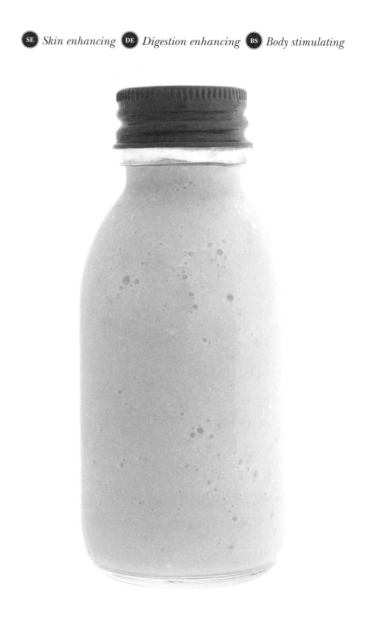

WATERCRESS

Slightly sweet

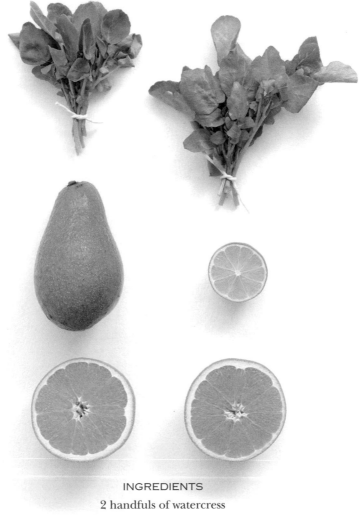

INGREDIENTS

2 handfuls of watercress

1 orange • 1 avocado

½ lime

Blend the ingredients. Add more water, if necessary,
to reach your desired consistency, then drink

This smoothie is full of vitamins A, C and K, and can also help to reduce early signs of a headache.

BN *Blood nourishing* **SE** *Skin enhancing* **A** *Alkalising*

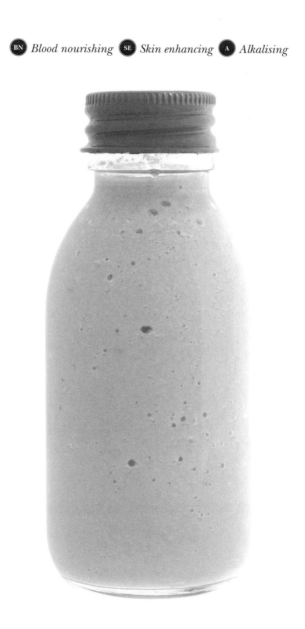

SKIN TONIC

Slightly sweet

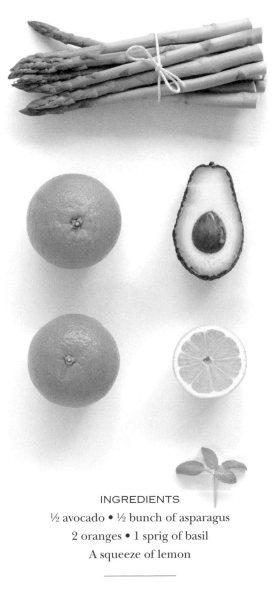

INGREDIENTS

½ avocado • ½ bunch of asparagus

2 oranges • 1 sprig of basil

A squeeze of lemon

Blend the ingredients. Add more water, if necessary, to
reach your desired consistency, then drink.

132

This smoothie enhances your beauty from within
because it's high in nutrients and fibre.

BS *Body stimulating* **BN** *Blood nourishing* **SE** *Skin enhancing*

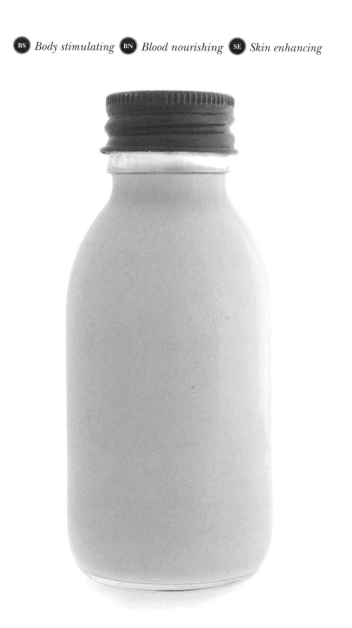

BLUEBERRY CHIA

Slightly sweet

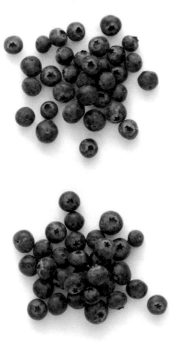

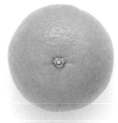

INGREDIENTS

2 handfuls of blueberries
1 orange • 1 tablespoon chia seeds
½ head of broccoli

Blend the ingredients. Add more water, if necessary, to
reach your desired consistency, then drink.

This smoothie is a natural aphrodisiac, aiding digestion
and helping to clear the mind.

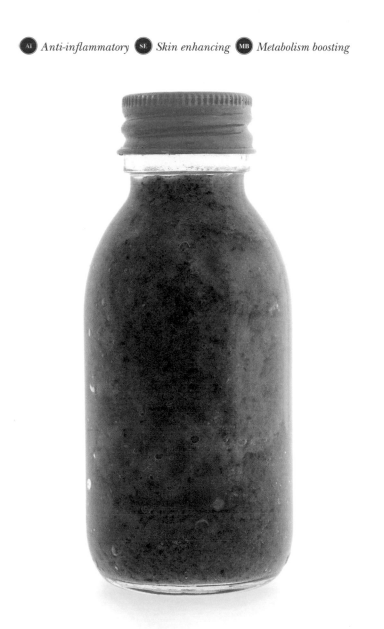 *Anti-inflammatory* 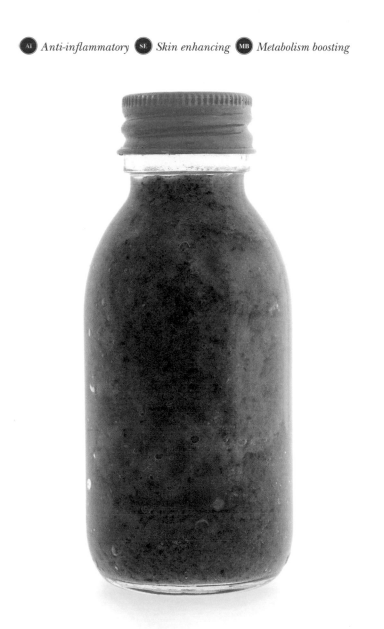 *Skin enhancing* 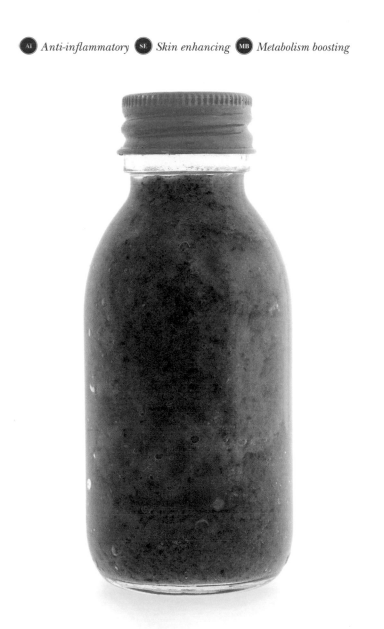 *Metabolism boosting*

SHOTS & MILKS

Shots are a great way of injecting some goodness into your diet when you need it. They can also be added to regular juices or smoothies for an extra pick-me-up. Milks are also highly nutritious. A natural sweetener is added to most milks, which can be increased according to taste. Popular sweeteners are agave syrup, raw honey, coconut oil and real maple syrup. All milks can been stored in the refrigerator for up to three days. Nuts are a vital part of all our diets because they are high in monounsaturated fats, which help keep our hearts healthy and disease free. They are also a great source of protein, minerals and other life-enhancing nutrients. Some nuts are best soaked first before adding to your blender.

ALOE

Slightly sweet

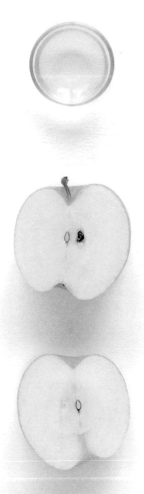

INGREDIENTS

1 teaspoon aloe vera juice

1 green apple, juiced

Pour the aloe vera juice into a glass, then stir in the juiced apple.

This shot helps to lower cholesterol and your blood sugar.

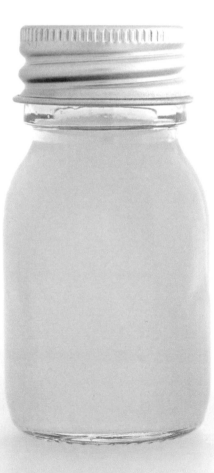 **BN** *Blood nourishing* **DE** *Digestion enhancing*

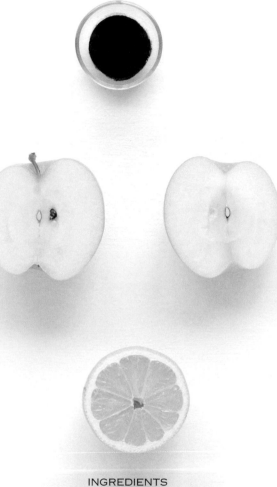

INGREDIENTS

1 teaspoon spirulina powder

1 green apple

A squeeze of lemon

Put the spirulina powder into a glass, then juice the apple and
add to the glass with the lemon juice. Combine well.

This shot is high in protein and minerals.

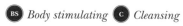 *Body stimulating* 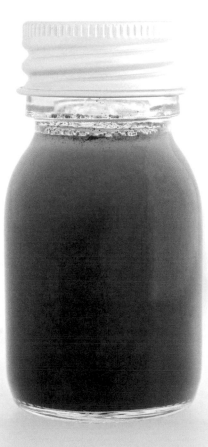 *Cleansing*

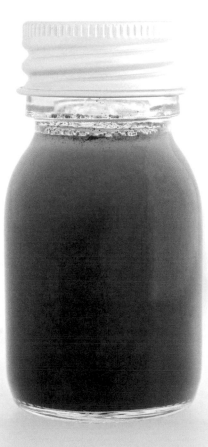

FLU KICK
Savoury

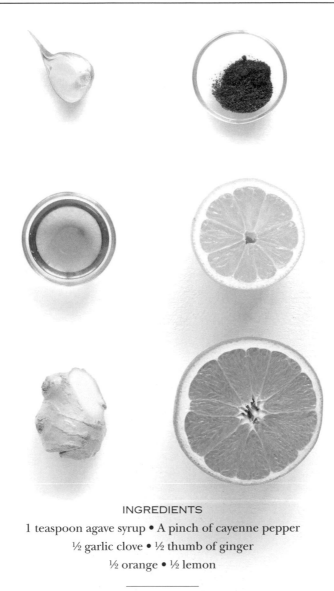

INGREDIENTS
1 teaspoon agave syrup • A pinch of cayenne pepper
½ garlic clove • ½ thumb of ginger
½ orange • ½ lemon

Put the agave syrup into a glass and add the cayenne. Juice the garlic, ginger,
orange and lemon, then pour into the glass. Not for the faint-hearted!

This shot provides a boost to your blood and will help to fight symptoms of the flu.

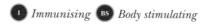 *Immunising* **BS** *Body stimulating*

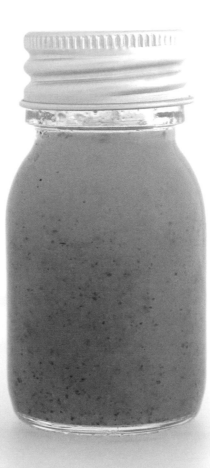

GINGER

Savoury

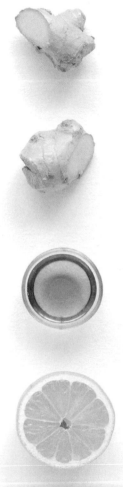

INGREDIENTS

1 teaspoon agave syrup

½ lemon

2 thumbs of ginger

Put the agave syrup into a glass, then juice the lemon and
ginger, and add to the glass. Combine well.

This shot is good for your respiratory system as well as your heart.

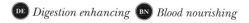 *Digestion enhancing* 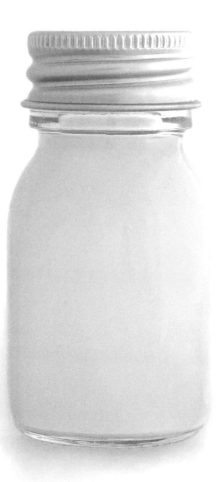 *Blood nourishing*

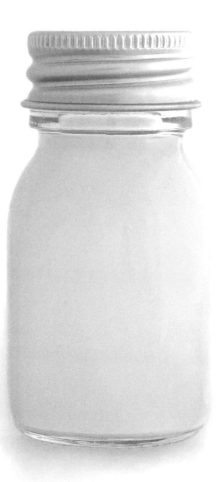

BRAZIL NUT MILK
Slightly sweet

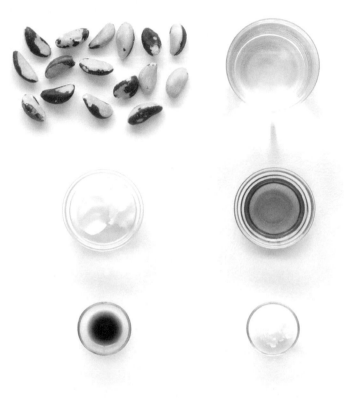

INGREDIENTS
150g brazil nuts • 2 tablespoons coconut oil

2 tablespoons agave syrup

1 teaspoon vanilla extract • A pinch of sea salt

Soak the brazil nuts in water for up to six hours to obtain the best flavour.
Dry the nuts before you start.

Place all the ingredients into a blender, together with 600ml water, and blend
for at least one minute. For best results, strain through a cheesecloth or a piece
of muslin, using a ladle to push through as much liquid as possible.

This special milk is full of fibre, selenium and vitamin E.

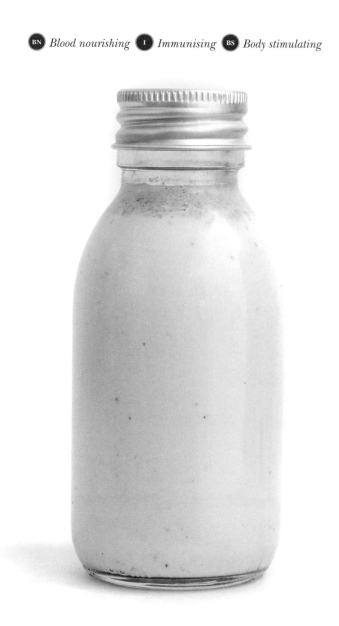 **BN** *Blood nourishing* **I** *Immunising* **BS** *Body stimulating*

PINE NUT MILK

Rich and sweet

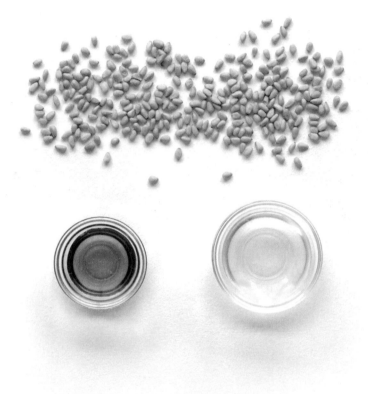

INGREDIENTS

75g pine nuts

2 tablespoons honey

Pine nuts do not need to be soaked.

Place the ingredients into a blender, together with 250ml water and whizz for a
good minute. Strain through a cheesecloth or a piece of muslin, using a ladle
to push through as much liquid as possible.

This is a delicious milk, which is rich in vitamin A and is also good for your heart.

I *Immunising* **FF** *Fat flushing*

ALMOND MILK
Slightly sweet

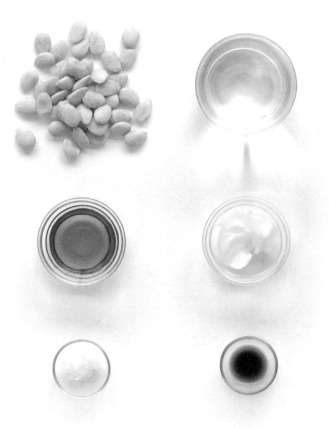

INGREDIENTS

150g almonds, soaked and drained

2 tablepoons coconut oil • 2 tablepoons agave syrup

1 teaspoon vanilla extract • A pinch of salt

For best results, soak your almonds for six to eight hours.

Blend the ingredients together with 600ml water until smooth and creamy.
Strain the liquid through a cheesecloth or muslin, using a ladle to push
through as much liquid as possible.

This is a great milk for lowering your cholesterol.

MBB *Muscle & bone building*   **AO** *Anti-oxidising*

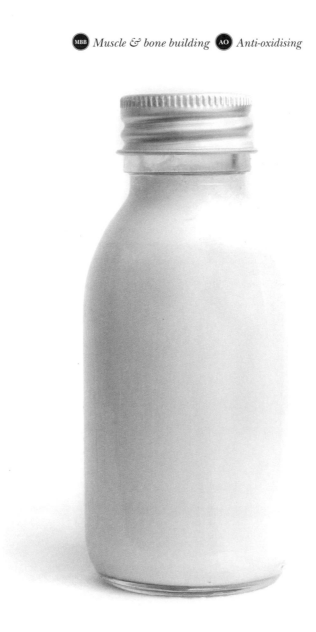

PUMPKIN SEED MILK

Slightly sweet

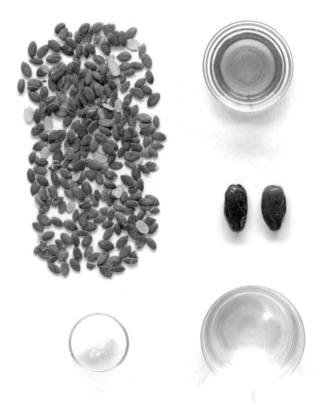

INGREDIENTS

125g pumpkin seeds

2 dates • 2 tablespoons honey

A pinch of salt

Blend all the ingredients together with 500ml water.
Strain the liquid through a cheesecloth or a piece of muslin, using a ladle
to push through as much liquid as possible.

A rich source of zinc, this milk helps you to sleep well and enhances your mood.

(A) *Alkalising* (AI) *Anti-inflammatory*

CHOCOLATE & CASHEW

Slightly sweet

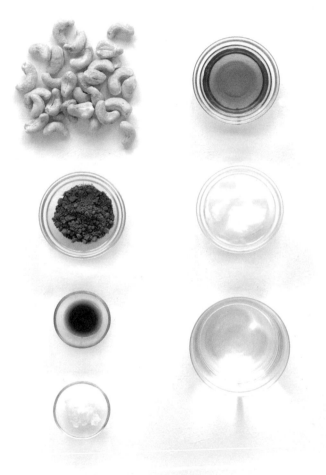

INGREDIENTS

100g cashew nuts • 30g cocoa powder
1 tablespoon coconut oil • 2 tablespoons agave syrup
1 teaspoon vanilla extract • ½ teaspoon salt

Blend all the ingredients together with 600ml water on high speed. Chill before
serving. If you would like this a little sweeter just add more agave syrup.

A protein-packed milk, which is a great mood enhancer.

I *Immunising* **AI** *Anti-inflammatory* **BN** *Blood nourishing*

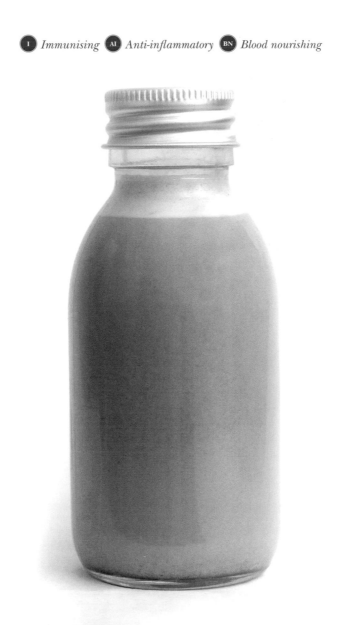

MILKY PECAN

Slightly sweet

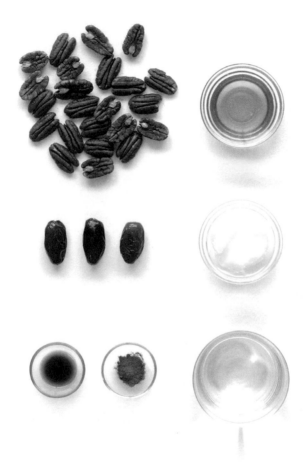

INGREDIENTS

115g pecans, toasted or unsalted

3 dates • 2 tablespoons agave syrup • 1 tablespoon coconut oil

1½ teaspoons ground cinnamon • ½ teaspoon vanilla extract

Soak pecans overnight or for six to eight hours for best results.
Place all the ingredients into a blender together with 360ml water and blend
for at least one minute. Chill before drinking.

This milk contains over 20 essential vitamins and minerals.

BN *Blood nourishing* **DE** *Digestion enhancing* **BP** *Brain powering*

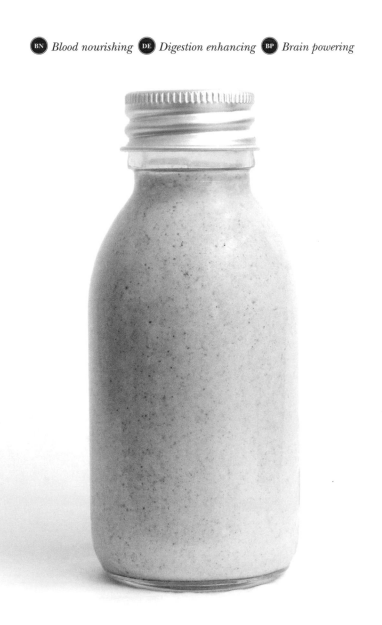

INDEX

ACKNOWLEDGEMENTS

THANK YOU M AND M

An Hachette UK Company | www.hachette.co.uk

First published in Great Britain in 2015 by
Hamlyn, a division of Octopus Publishing Group Ltd
Carmelite House, 50 Victoria Embankment,
London EC4Y 0DZ
www.octopusbooks.co.uk

Originally published by Marabout, 43 Quai de Grenelle, 75905 Paris, CEDEX 15

Copyright © Hachette Livre (Marabout) 2014

Copyright this English-language edition © Hachette Livre (Marabout) 2015

All rights reserved. No part of this work may be reproduced or utilized in any form or by any means, electronic or mechanical, including photocopying, recording or by any information storage and retrieval system, without the prior written permission of the publisher.

Fern Green asserts the moral right to be identified as the author of this work.

ISBN 978-0-600-63208-5

A CIP catalogue record for this book is available from the British Library.

Printed and bound in China.

3 5 7 9 10 8 6 4 2

Senior Editor: Leanne Bryan
Senior Art Editor: Juliette Norsworthy
Designer: Helen McTeer
Photographer: Deirdre Rooney
Assistant Production Manager: Caroline Alberti

For further information about the blenders and juicers mentioned in this book, go to:

www.vitamix.com

www.blendtec.com

www.pro-juice.co.uk

www.magimix.com

www.omegajuicers.com

www.ukjuicers.com